"Caroline is one of the most inspiring people I have ever met. She lights up the room, and people are naturally drawn to her positive attitude. Her energy is contagious. The world needs more Caroline Jordan."

—Sarah Clifford Kaney, friend, class participant, recruiting lead in finance

"Wherever you are in your fitness goals, Caroline meets you there and shows you how far you can go. Whether you're on a bike, a plane, or a conference call, she knows how to keep your body happy, healthy, and hungry for more challenges. Above all, she inspires you to be grateful for your health, to love your body, and to strive to reach your full potential."

—Mia Campitelli, friend and coaching client

"Caroline's positive energy and passion for fitness are infectious! She truly has a gift for helping people establish their own health and wellness plan as well as providing the tools in order for people to be their best, happy self!"

—Jennifer Glatzer, occupational therapist at Stanford

"Caroline's energy and passion for fitness are contagious. She has a gift for helping people use health as a platform to achieve every life goal."

—Lisa Kant, friend and coaching client

"Caroline's positive outlook on fitness has me viewing workouts as something good for my body and mind, rather than something I have to do to burn off dessert or look better on the beach. Caroline taught me that fitness is not about what your body looks like—it's about what your body can do. The immense joy she exudes as my fitness coach has in turn made me stronger, fitter, and feeling great both inside and out."

—Sally French, coaching client and
digital editor, Dow Jones Media Group

"Caroline doesn't know me, and I don't know her, and although that is true, she is one of my best friends. She finds me 'virtually' whenever I need a pick-me-up or a little extra motivation. Her super-cheery disposition and attitude to health and happiness spread joy far beyond those who have the pleasure of being with her in person."

—Eva Wisenbeck, YouTube subscriber

"Caroline Jordan is the epitome of inspirational: she is genuine, cheerful, encouraging, deliberate, passionate, and more enthusiastic than several people I know combined. She is truly a bright spot in the fitness and wellness community, inspiring people to do more, be more, and live more while pursuing health, happiness, and wellness. Caroline is one of the most authentic people I have had the pleasure of knowing, and she genuinely cares about her world and the people in it, while also striving to carve out her place and make her mark. This unique balance is truly remarkable."

—Jennifer Kirchhofer, friend, fan, class participant,
and marketing professional

"Caroline Jordan always carries herself with positive energy and a can-do attitude. This is why I keep coming back to her for fitness guidance."

—Naomi Han, RN and coaching client

"In her weekly group fitness classes, Caroline has taught me to find happiness in tough situations. It is happiness that lasts beyond class time and does more than make me smile—it empowers me to internalize positive messages that quite simply enable me to tackle difficult issues, increasingly stronger each time. Caroline shares the positivity and supplies the tools for you to upgrade your own life. That makes her encouraging, nonjudgmental of others' paths toward optimism, and surely worth following as long as she keeps teaching."

—Sabrina Kippur, MS, certified Pilates instructor

"Caroline embodies all that is inspiration. After knowing her from a fitness angle from various workout classes and using her as a consultant for a charity running team, I had the privilege of hosting Caroline at the Junior League of San Francisco as a speaker for a training and development course. Caroline spoke not just about how to keep your body healthy but also about how to achieve your goals, both personal and professional, by laying out a plan and applying smart tactics. She is a true lifestyle guru who is able to break down goals, problems, and issues into achievable steps to help you become the person you want to be. The thirty-plus attendees left inspired and ready to take on the new year with style and elegance, just like Caroline herself! Should you have the opportunity to work with Caroline, or have her speak at an event, I wouldn't pass it up—she will set you on the path to being the best version of yourself."

—Kelly Keele, Assistant Director of Prospect Research, Stanford University

"This girl rocks. Her enthusiasm for life and fitness is contagious, and she always has a smile and a kind, encouraging word to offer. All around, Caroline is an awesome person and an awesome inspiration."

—Heather S, wellness client

"Caroline has been an inspiration to me for the ten-plus years that I have been a member at Equinox. She is always smiling and enthusiastic. Her disposition is always sunny, and it is genuine. She practices what she preaches in the way she lives her life. She is a pleasure to work with and definitely gives you your money's worth."

—Nancy Raabe, class participant and community member

"Caroline Jordan has endless valuable tools and tips that are easy to implement and that make a difference. Her infectious enthusiasm and passion for living a better life will keep you coming back for more."

—Hal Rosenberg, DC, CCSP, Sports Chiropractic

"Within the first month of working with Caroline, my mental strength reached a whole new level of fitness. Thank you, Caroline, for all your positivity and strength week after week, day after day."

—Katie McKernan, coaching client

"Caroline: Thank you, thank you, thank you for being a positive influence in my life! Each day I have a moment with you in it to remind me to live life in love, either sweating in spin class or reading your Sunday newsletter, is a lucky day! Your positive attitude and spirit help me through long days at work, or whatever else I'm getting through at the moment, to remind me to take time for myself."

—Rose Kelly, fitness class participant
and community member

"'POSITIVE ENERGY. POSITIVE RESULTS.' With that strong and truthful philosophy, Caroline Jordan has captivated my mind and heart. Caroline is truly living her positive philosophy and is inspiring, fascinating, and motivating people. She is an excellent teacher and coach with a magnetic quality to pull out the magnificence in people. She enables people to fulfill their dreams and to reach their goals, and she shows you the most important ways to feel energized and to create a mind and a body to love yourself. In her cooperative workshops she provides the key steps for a better work-life balance and helps you understand how to increase your quality of life. She has great charisma, she's infectiously good-humored, and she spreads happiness and joy. Of course, there are also bad days and times in a person's life, but in these phases she also nimbly accepts the current situation, but she doesn't allow negative thoughts to pull her down. There is always a solution, and everything happens for a reason. She helps you to find out and to strengthen your access to your mental and physical self."

—Anna Kemph, health and wellness coach and colleague

BALANCED BODY
BREAKTHROUGH

BALANCED BODY BREAKTHROUGH

Get Your Mind, Body, and Spirit
in Great Shape So You Can Love Your Life

Caroline Jordan

Published by Quill, an imprint of Inkshares, Inc., San Francisco, California
www.inkshares.com

Cover design by Lexie Tiongson
Interior photos © Kuroda Studios

ISBN: 9781942645115
e-ISBN: 9781942645542
Library of Congress Control Number: 2016935639

First edition

Printed in the United States of America

To my mother, who taught me how and showed me the way. To my father, who is my rock and my eternal source of sunshine. To my brother and his wife, who show me how to love and live fully. Thank you. I love you. I will celebrate the incredible family that you are today and always.

CONTENTS

PREFACE

Through my work in wellness, I see many people struggle to find balance, health, and self-care in their lives. Burnout and stress are a growing epidemic that is making our world sick, tired, and joyless. Burnout—the mental and physical exhaustion you experience when the demands of your life consistently exceed the amount of energy you have available—has been called the illness of the modern world. We are seeing alarming increases in mental and physical diseases caused or exacerbated by stress. One in two men and one in three women are projected to develop cancer in their lifetime. Forty million adults in the United States suffer from anxiety disorders. In addition, 47 percent of US physicians report at least one symptom of burnout.

One thing I know for sure: killing yourself through overwork is not going to help you succeed. Think of how you feel after a poor night's sleep or how you feel when you go too long without a nutritious meal. If your health fails, your performance in your life does too. It's all backward. Your health needs to be number one if you want to be your best.

It's time to stop working harder and start working smarter. My goal has been to make this book a source of inspiration, information, encouragement, and support to help readers personalize their approach to balance and find health. The resources in this book are real, tested, and ready to powerfully impact the reader's life. Much of the content from the book is material I present at wellness workshops, lectures, special events, presentations, classes, and coaching sessions. I see the material work magic, and it's been so well received that I wanted to put it in one place. I truly believe in this book's content and I am positive that it will inspire both individual and community wellness.

The introduction is my own personal story: how I recovered from burnout and became the balanced wellness coach I am today. It describes my why and how I want to help the reader in living a healthy, happy life. Chapter 1 is an in-depth coaching exercise designed to help readers define their ideal vision of success and set SMART goals to take action steps forward. The body, mind, and spirit chapters that follow are full of resources, strategies, and tools that can be used individually or together to accomplish readers' goals and their personal vision of wellness.

Defining what you want to accomplish, combined with customizing a program tailored to your needs, will help you move forward in achieving your ideal vision of health. Everybody's body and athletic preferences are different. This book is designed as a guide to help readers personalize their approach to living well and empower them to take real action toward achieving their definition of success.

I invite you to take a deep breath and think about your life. Are you moving forward in the direction you want? Deep down, what is truly important to you? What do you value, and do you make time for it on a daily basis? My goal is to be a source of inspiration, information, encouragement, and support to enable you to take action and live a life you love. Start now. This book is a tool. Set small, realistic goals to make those things that truly matter to you a part of your world. Whether you are trying to beat stress, have specific fitness feats you want to accomplish, or want to take better care of yourself, I'm here to help you keep your body, mind, and spirit in great shape so you can love your life.

Remember: Success is not the key to happiness. Happiness is the key to success. I believe in you and I believe you have the power to choose to love yourself and love your life. And if ever you forget your own greatness, I want to be the voice that's there to remind you of your strength. Stay committed, positive, present, and persistent. You deserve to feel good and to live a life you love.

Keep going, keep growing, and get ready to make your happiness happen.

Caroline

INTRODUCTION

The Modern Hero's Journey:
From Burnout to Balance

Have you ever been so chronically tired that you just can't seem to think straight? Your emotions are all over the map, and you get easily upset? Or you feel resentful, jealous, maybe even angry with the people in your life? Do you feel overwhelmed most of the time? Weighed down with stress, overcommitted, spread too thin? Have you ever experienced random aches and pains, suffered from inexplicable weight loss or gain, or gotten sick far too often? You try to think positively, but you just can't seem to get out of the funk. You are burned out. And it's time to take care of yourself.

I know this place well. I was in chronic burnout mode all of 2010. Moody, anxious, frazzled, filled with self-doubt. In this state, your mind shuts off. You are going through the motions, doing what's expected of you, and not fully experiencing life. I knew this wasn't the way I wanted to live, but I was too tired to fix it. The only solution I knew was to work harder—I didn't know a way out. Since my mind wasn't in the right place, I listened to the needs and wants of everyone else. It was as if I was living my life on autopilot. It took a major wake-up call to snap me out of it. Life was meant for so much more than eat, sleep, work, repeat.

My breakthrough moment is a vivid memory. It was the end of 2011, and I collapsed on my San Francisco studio floor. I was exhausted. I had the career I thought I wanted, yet I had wrecked my life in the process. I was a mental, emotional, and physical mess with no energy left to live my life.

I spent my days working. In the evenings I rested. That was about it. Work. Rest. Work. Rest. I didn't have energy for anything else. While on the outside it looked like I had it together, inside I was falling apart. It wasn't rock bottom—I had many things in my life to be grateful for. But I was too tired to appreciate them and felt completely disconnected from myself and my world. I was seeking love and self-worth through my work. The unfortunate part was that work didn't love me back.

Don't get me wrong: I did this to myself. When I was fifteen, my big dream was to become "America's next top fitness instructor." I worked endlessly to climb the ladder, to build my brand, to look the part, and to fit in the box of what was seen as successful. I hustled hard, put myself last, and did what I thought I had to do to succeed. I was good at my job and loved helping others but I was putting the rest of my life on hold and hurting myself in the process. I didn't know my own worth, didn't love myself, and was looking for love everywhere else. The truth is that helping others and being a career success doesn't help you love yourself. You've got to love yourself first.

I knew I was at a crossroads. I had a choice: continue to do what wasn't working or change my life. I made a choice and paused everything. It was time to face the truth, get real, and restart. I had built a career based on what I thought the world wanted, but what did I want for myself? I started from the foundation: learn to love yourself. Then I rebuilt my life based on my own definition of success.

That moment was the catalyst that catapulted my life in a different direction. I declared 2012 the "Year of Self-Love" and every day chose to take action toward loving myself from within. It was scary at first. I didn't know how to start. So I hired coaches, read books, and created vision boards. I made time for my physical health through consistent workouts, nourishing meals, and rest. I invested in myself and went back to school to become a health and wellness coach. A lot can happen when you want it to. I healed through self-discovery, self-love, and living life according to my own vision of success and how I wanted to positively impact the world.

One thing I know for sure: learning to love yourself will be the hardest thing you'll ever do. But you're worth it—so worth it. And you can change your world.

Through this process, I got my life back. I gained balance, confidence, energy, strength, and health. From this authentic, grounded place I became a success and my career followed. (Yes, imagine how that works!) The cliché is true: Self-love is the number one key to success.

Making a living is not the same as making a life. I'm proud of myself for working hard to build happiness in both.

My story is not uncommon. In fact, in today's world it's starting to become the norm. We love the idea of others loving us, and we forget to love ourselves. We look for love outside ourselves through our career accomplishments, relationships, achievements, fitness, clothes, and material items. But no amount of success, fame, or love from someone else can fill a void created by a lack of self-love. Love is an inside job, and in order to receive it we have to already have it within.

It's time to learn to be your own best friend instead of falling into the trap of being your own worst enemy. Are you ready to be your number-one priority and take action in living a life you love? Wellness is something that you deserve to have in your life. It is something worth working for every day and enables you to live fully. Nothing is worth it if you aren't happy or healthy. You were given this one life to live, and your health and happiness are priceless.

Have you ever lost your balance? Do you struggle to juggle the important priorities in your life? Have you ever lost your sense of self while working to accomplish your goals? Do you have a hard time putting yourself first or practicing self-care? Did you have a breakthrough, or are you looking to have one now?

This book holds the tools I used to transform my life, to help you take care of yourself so you can be a success inside and out. If you want to value your life, you have to be willing to fight for your health and happiness. Are you ready to have a breakthrough? Are you ready to work hard for you?

Our world provides plenty of signals telling us to push harder and climb higher up the ladder, but there are almost no signals reminding us to stay connected to who we are, to take care of ourselves, and to lead fulfilling lives. I want to be that voice that empowers you: Live this life for you. Create your world according to your own definition of success and thrive with more health, more joy, more love, and more gratitude.

It was a great blessing to hit burnout; that moment was a wake-up call that forever changed my course. It led me back to myself and opened my eyes to a new way of life. It connected me to my purpose: to be the change and empower a healthier, happier planet.

Right now you may feel busy, stressed, overwhelmed, and exhausted. I've been there and know exactly how you feel! But if you want to have a breakthrough, you have to make time for yourself. This book will help guide you to do just that.

Here's our plan of action to enable you to beat burnout and find balance: Chapter 1 is an essential step that will help you better understand who you are, know what you want, and define a clear wellness vision. It will take you step by step through creating a personalized action plan to get you where you want to go and to aid you in realizing your greatest potential. I'm inviting you to get honest, get specific, and take back control of your life. The Body, Mind, and Spirit sections (chapters 2 through 11) are full of resources, strategies, and tools that help you achieve your wellness vision and the goals you set in Chapter 1. The resources from each chapter can be used individually or together to help you accomplish the thriving life your heart desires. Think of it like a lifestyle buffet: you fill your plate with the suggestions and strategies that work for you. It might sound like a lot of work right now, but don't worry—I'll be your coach through the process, asking you questions and guiding you to continue to customize your lifestyle based on your wants and needs. What you read here and what you choose to do with it can help you beat burnout by personalizing your approach to living well and empowering you to take real action toward achieving your vision of life success.

Living a balanced life is an evolving process and a constant work in progress. Remember to give yourself permission to move at your own pace. What matters most is that you commit to making time for yourself and taking intentional, consistent actions toward your goals. You can't do this without you. You are the hero of your story, and I'm here to support you 110 percent. It won't be easy, and it won't transpire overnight, but it is possible. The process begins when you decide that there has to be a better way to live and that you deserve to discover it.

PART I
Vision

If you don't know where you are going, you'll probably end up somewhere else.
—*Laurence J. Peter*

Does it ever feel like you work hard but don't seem to get anywhere worthwhile? It could be because you haven't spent enough time thinking about what you want from life or setting formal goals for yourself. After all, would you set out on a major journey with no real idea of your destination? Probably not!

Vision-defining and goal-setting exercises are powerful practices for motivating you to turn your ideal future into reality. By knowing precisely what you want to achieve, you know where you want to concentrate your efforts. Defining a vision and setting goals help you choose where you want to go in life.

The problem is that when most people are looking to make a lifestyle change or accomplish a goal, they follow a cookie-cutter program or a supposedly quick-fix solution like a "30-Day Diet," "Fit in 5," or "10 Days to Calm." While these approaches might work temporarily, they are not sustainable long term or customized to meet your unique needs. Balanced living is not a quick fix—it's a lifestyle. Your balanced lifestyle is something you need to design and find for yourself. I want to give you the tools that can help you personalize your own program. I believe that by defining your vision and completing goal-setting exercises you'll be able to customize your own approach to balanced living that works with your life and for your life.

The exercises in this chapter are designed to help guide you in defining, discovering, and designing your own vision for success and crafting a unique strategy for achieving your goals and lasting results. They can be reused anytime you and your lifestyle goals change. Each exercise will help you cook up your own personalized recipe for success and set you up with a smart action plan to start moving forward. I encourage you to revisit these helpful planning tools often as you evolve and continue to define goals you'd like to work toward.

These vision and goal exercises were complete game changers for me in recovering from burnout, getting to know myself, and developing goals that produced real results. With their help, I got honest with myself about what I needed to do to live a balanced life. Then I set clearly defined goals and took action toward my ideal vision of balance. Others commented about the change: "Caroline you are glowing. It looks like everything is going well! You look so happy, what have you been doing?" It was simple: I had spent time asking myself who I was and how I wanted to live. Then, from my truth, I set smart goals and took action toward making my vision happen.

If you don't know who you are, what you want, and how to accomplish it, you'll get lost or experience even more burnout.

Some of the exercises may seem obvious or basic to you, but if you really want to beat burnout you need to take the time, have an open mind, and do the work. Many people are so eager to get started that they skip this essential piece, head straight into action, make it extreme, fizzle out fast, and are left back where they started (or worse). Don't let that be you. Roll up your sleeves, spend some quality time with yourself, and get real. Ask yourself what matters to you and how you want to live your life. Do the work. You'll be infinitely more successful if you create a compelling vision, set goals, get support, and take focused action to move forward toward real results.

Do not press Go until you've worked through the exercises. Make time for them, and you'll see amazing results. YOU are your secret to success!

CHAPTER 1
Secrets for Success

CREATING A CLEAR VISION

To get going, you need to define exactly where you are and where you want to go. To begin, define your starting point. Don't censor yourself and be honest. Remember: this is for you. Set a timer for 10 minutes and free-write your answers to the following questions.

Where Am I Now?

- How do I feel overall right now?
- How do I feel about:
    - my fitness?
    - my relationships?
    - my career?
    - my finances?
    - my spiritual life?
    - the way I look?

- How do I feel about the overall quality of my life?
- What frustrates me most about my health, fitness, and nutrition habits?
- How long has it been since I've had fun and adventure?
- And most important: What would I like to change?

Great job! I know that was tough, maybe even emotional. I'm proud of you for taking the time, working through the exercise, and defining your starting point. Now it's time to clarify what you want to achieve and to create a detailed vision statement.

Where Do I Want to Go?

A vision statement is a description of yourself in the future and the health-promoting, life-giving behaviors you see yourself doing consistently. Write your vision statement now. Define where you'd like to go and what you'd like to do. Create a clear, descriptive vision of what your idea of success looks like. Include health, fitness, relationships, career, finances, hobbies, and all elements that make your ideal vision compelling, motivational, and personal. Write down how you see your ideal life. Write and write and write some more. Set a timer for 10 minutes and describe in detail what your ideal life looks like. If you go over 10 minutes, that's okay. Reminder: don't censor yourself; be honest.

- How do I feel overall?
- How do I feel about:
    my relationships?
    my career?
    my finances?
    my spiritual life?

- How is my health?
- How many times a week do I exercise?
- What is my diet like?
- What do I look like?
- How many times a week do I see friends?
- How is my mind-set?
- What is my mood like?
- How is the quality of my life overall?
- What do I do for fun and adventure?
- What changes have I made?
- What goals have I accomplished?
- What am I most proud of?

MOVING AHEAD

Don't get overwhelmed if your vision feels far off or out of reach right now. To help simplify, let's break it down into key elements, core values, motivators, challenges, strengths, and supports. Set a timer for each section, and write!

Key Elements

- What are the most important elements in your vision?
- Are there specific themes in terms of health, relationships, fitness, spirituality, and so on?

Core Values

Aim for listing at least three top values that you want to prioritize.

- Without being modest, what do you value most about your life?
- What values does your vision support?
- Are these values priorities in your life right now? Do you want them to be?

Motivators

Write down at least three factors that motivate you to do the work needed to realize your vision.

- What makes this vision important to you?
- Why do you want to achieve this vision?
- What good will come from doing so?
- Why do you want to achieve this outcome?

Challenges

Write down challenges or obstacles you see that might come between you and achieving your vision.

- What obstacles or challenges are limiting your life potential?
- What significant events do you anticipate having to deal with on the way to reaching your vision?
- What concerns you most?
- What do you see affecting your ability to achieve your vision?
- What are possible strategies you could use to overcome these obstacles?
- Thinking outside the box, how can you be your own hero?

Strengths

- What character strengths can you draw on to help you realize your vision and meet your challenges?
- How can the lessons from your past successes in life carry over to your current challenges?
- Are you using your strengths to live your most powerful life?

If you'd like to dive deeper, you can identify your signature strengths by taking the Values-in-Action (VIA) Signature Strengths questionnaire. This is one of the most popular surveys in the world and is available (for free) online. To date more than 1.8 million people have registered on the website and taken the tests and between 500 and 1,500 new people register every day. This questionnaire identifies 24 character strengths, grouped into six large categories called virtues that consistently emerge across history and culture.

Knowing your constellation of signature character strengths can help you toward living a happier, more authentic life. Take the free test and pay attention to the rank order of your strengths. Were there any surprises for you? How can you use these strengths to help you achieve your vision and goals?

Supports

- What people, resources, systems, and environments can you draw on to help you realize your vision and overcome challenges?
- How can you use your strengths, environments, or relationships to overcome obstacles to your well being success?

Once you've made a list, reconnect with at least three people, resources, or systems that you believe will help you realize your vision. When it comes to wellness and balance, people are generally accountable only to themselves and often that isn't enough. Building in accountability and real support helps ensure that you will remain on track. Here are a few examples:

- Call a friend and tell them about your vision. Ask for their encouragement, support, and help.
- Connect with a gym and register for a weekly workout class. Get motivation and accountability from signing up and working out with a group.
- Invest in online nutrition coaching, and use the website's system of weekly menu plans and healthy recipes to help guide you in healthy eating. Stay on track by using this resource to help you accomplish your healthy diet habits.

DEFINE, DESIGN, COMMIT, SUCCEED

Congratulations! You did it! You took the time to figure out your unique vision, identify your strengths, and get clear on what you want to accomplish. This is the beginning of a healthier, happier you. I know that takes a lot of work, and I want you to be proud of yourself. Now that you have designed your motivating well-being vision, how ready, confident, and committed are you to take the next steps?

Keeping your goal in mind, let's work together to set goals that will help you create a plan of action. The next step is to complete a few more exercises to help you get "started smart." You can do it!

SMART GOALS

Are you feeling motivated by your wellness vision? Great! Just remember that motivation alone is not enough to get you there. Without a clear plan of action, motivation will fade in the face of challenge. Your next step is to set SMART goals.

Goals make visions real. They help you define a clear path that leads to making your vision a reality. In order to work, your balanced body goals need to be SMART:

S	Specific (or Significant)
M	Measurable (or Meaningful)
A	Attainable (or Action Oriented)
R	Relevant (or Rewarding)
T	Time Bound (or Trackable)

Using this method to state your goals puts you fully in charge of accomplishing your vision through completing specific, measurable, realistic steps. Being realistic is essential in setting yourself up for long-term progress. Nothing hurts the change process or your self-esteem more than setting unrealistic, unachievable goals.

When helping clients set goals using the SMART method, I always tell them to act like a news reporter. If your goal was on the news, what would be the who, what, when, where, and why? Cover all the bases when defining and describing your goal.

Compare the following statements and consider which statement sounds more actionable to you:

Goal: "I want to develop a strength routine to be strong and healthy."

SMART goal: "I will complete a strength routine using 10 to 20 exercises, targeting all my major muscle groups, for 20 minutes at least twice a week."

Goal: "I will be less stressed."
SMART goal: "Every workday at 3:00 p.m. I will take a regular break to get outside, go for a walk, and de-stress."

Goal: "I will eat healthier meals."
SMART goal: "I will make a grocery list and shop every Saturday morning for at least five days of meals and snacks per week." Or "I will use eatingwell.com for meal plans, grocery lists, recipes, and guides."

SMART goals help you to create achievable little steps and mini successes. This will keep you motivated as you move forward toward your vision. Great things take time, consistent effort, focused action, and a lot of patience. Remember: "Rome wasn't built in a day." As Epictetus would say, "No great thing is created suddenly." Take one small step at a time. Be positive and persistent. Combine your wellness vision with SMART goal setting, and you will be ready to take action and be a success!

REFINING YOUR VISION

Here are a few examples of visions, divided into three-month goals and weekly goals.

Sample Vision 1: Haley, Age 32

My vision is that I am more organized, healthier, leaner, and more energetic. I am 10 pounds lighter, and I glow because I am healthy and eating right. I love to wake up and run or spin every morning—it makes my day! Because I wake up early, I don't have to leave during work and can get more done during the day. I make healthy meals for myself and bring them for lunch four days per week.

My primary motivators are to feel more confident, be disciplined with my time, and feel healthier.

My strengths are my competitiveness and determination to hit my goals.

My main current pattern is that I sway back and forth from routine, and when I fall off I fall hard. I lose my diet regime, my workout schedule, and control. I sleep in late, have to leave work to exercise, and have a glass of wine for no reason.

My strategy to outgrow this pattern is to start by setting a schedule every morning, starting with the time I wake up; getting in exercise; taking vitamins; watching my diet; and limiting wine to social events.

Three-Month Goals: Haley, Age 32

Month Started: August 2015

Fitness Goal: I will work out 6 days each week for 35 to 60 minutes. I will increase my endurance to run 6 miles straight. Comments: go for a run, spin class, group fitness, hiking outside.

Nutrition Goal: I will set a vitamin routine and meal prep for workday lunches. I will use Sunday evening to prepare my lunches for the workweek.

Schedule: I will wake up by 6:00 a.m. every weekday morning to start my day with a workout. On weekends, I will wakeup by 7:30 a.m. to start my day with a workout.

Weight Goal: I will lose 10 to 15 pounds by following my new schedule of fitness and a healthy diet. Comments: weigh in Sunday and Wednesday each week and make a chart. Keep track of praise and why I successfully completed the week. Hold myself responsible.

This Week's Goals: Haley, Age 32

Week 1: Starting August 9

Fitness Goal: Go for two 2-mile jogs. Record my time and distance. Make a note if I needed to stop. Go to two spin classes at Equinox. Do two 30-minute strength workouts.

Nutrition Goal: Start by taking a daily women's vitamin and biotin. Look into healthy doses of vitamins D, E, and B. Make sure I'm getting enough of those. Learn about the nutrition I need to feel my best.

Weight Goal: Record my weight on Sunday as the starting weight. Weigh myself again on Wednesday.

Schedule Goal: Start waking up at 6:00 a.m. every day and get up. Comments: go for a short jog or just get out and get some fresh air to wake up.

Sample Vision 2: Megan, Age 40

My vision is that I am energetic, relaxed, and fit. I am 10 pounds lighter and glowing with health. I work out 4 to 5 times a week and eat nutritious meals that fuel me. I am managing stress better and spend 2 to 4 nights socializing with others.

My primary motivators are to feel more confident, in control, and to like myself more.

My strengths are my determination and persistence, which I use consistently for work and less consistently for self-care.

My main current pattern is that in periods of higher stress I tend to eat sugary snacks and lose my motivation to stay on track with my plan to lose weight.

My strategy to outgrow this pattern is to decrease mindless eating by taking a break from what I am doing and either go for a short walk or take a few minutes for meditation.

Three-Month Goals: Megan, Age 40

Month Started: September 2012

Fitness Goal: I will do a workout 3 days per week for 30 to 45 minutes. Comments: go for a run outside, take spin class, or go to group fitness classes

Nutrition Goal: I will eat 3 to 4 fruits, 5 days each week. Comments: fruit will replace sugary snacks.

Stress Goal: I will practice meditation for 20 minutes, 3 days each week. Comments: reduce my average daily stress rating (at the end of the workday when I feel most stressed) from 7 out of 10 to less than 5 and use the Jon Kabat-Zinn meditation program.

Weight Goal: I will lose 5 to 10 pounds by following my fitness and nutrition goals. Comments: weigh in weekly to chart progress and work with a personal trainer to adjust plan if needed.

This Week's Goals: Megan, Age 40

Week 1: Starting September 5

Fitness Goal: Run 3-mile loop around the local lake on Monday and Wednesday mornings. Comments: record my runs in Runkeeper app to track my time.

Nutrition Goal: Review list of fruits and check off those I would want to eat as a snack. Comments: may purchase a few on weekly visit to store.

Weight Goal: Weigh self next Tuesday and write weight in log. Comments: Track progress and share with my personal trainer.

Stress Goal: Do Jon Kabat-Zinn's 10-minute Lying Down Meditation on Sunday morning. Comments: Rate my stress level before and after on a scale of 1 to 10.

PUTTING IT ALL TOGETHER: GET GOING

Start with the end in mind. Take your wellness vision and divide it into three-month and weekly goals. Make each goal specific, measurable, actionable, realistic, and timed. Make it SMART!

You made it! I'm proud of you for working through the planning process and taking the time to set yourself up for success. Now that you've done the work, you have a clear path to get started toward a healthier, happier you. The next steps require action. Are you ready to make it happen?

In the following chapters, you'll learn effective ways to strengthen your body, mind, and spirit. Each section is full of tools, resources, and strategies that can be used individually or together to help you accomplish the goals you set in this chapter. It's a balanced body buffet! Choose the suggestions that work for you and fill your plate with what will help you accomplish your final vision.

PART II

Balanced Body

Beating burnout starts with taking care of your physical health. Mentally, physically, and emotionally, your life is in a better state when you are well. Taking the time to energize yourself with exercise, nourish yourself with good food, and ground yourself with rest is the recipe that allows you to be your best. I want you to look at your fitness as something you want to do to *feel* good, not just as something you should do to *look* good. Your energy and health are essential ingredients to your success.

The two biggest barriers that keep people from exercising and eating right are time and negative thinking about themselves. I'm here to help you move past those roadblocks. I offer you a chance to take action, to improve your self-esteem, and to be fit and happy inside and out. Remember: You have a choice. You are in control of beating burnout and choosing to live a balanced life. I know you have a lot to juggle and people who need you, but if your health fails you won't be able to do any of it. What kind of life would that be? Do you want to feel energetic, confident, powerful, balanced, and well? Then it's time to move your health to the top of your priority list. One of my main goals in writing this book is to encourage people to adopt a positive relationship to fitness and to feel good about themselves. I passionately believe that everyone deserves to feel healthy, be happy, and embrace life. We have so much to live for! I hope this will open a door to your future and help you live your life to the fullest.

This section is your go-to guide for enhancing your health through fitness, nutrition, rest, and time management. It will give you real resources to use in personalizing a solid balanced-body self-care program that works for you. It will help you learn how to take care of yourself when you feel like you don't have the time or energy. The tools in the following pages will give you the strength to overcome stress and live your best life.

CHAPTER 2

Fitness

I believe exercise is one of the most powerful ingredients in beating burnout and living a healthy life. When you move your body, you move your life. I want you to get moving. Get away from your desk, unplug from your smartphone, leave your to-do list at home, and take a break for yourself. Get your blood flowing and your heart pumping. Ignite your metabolism and build lean muscles that will make you powerful inside and out. You are worth every ounce of effort.

I wish I could tell you that exercising and beating burnout are easy, but you and I both know that's not true. There are no miracle cures or quick fixes, but it isn't overwhelmingly difficult or complicated either. I can guarantee you that getting up and getting moving is the most important decision you can make to improve your overall health and quality of life.

Exercise is proven to stimulate the release of endorphins, a chemical in the brain that is shown to be a natural antidepressant. All forms of movement prompt you to use muscles, which forces oxygen-rich blood to flow throughout the body and thereby increasing available energy. In addition, the stretching and contracting of muscles and tendons relieves stiffness, pain, and tension. The best part is that improving your physical health through exercise boosts your mental strength and confidence, enabling you to better manage life's challenges and live without burnout. Exercise is the best antidote to stress.

I invite you to stop looking at fitness as something you feel you should do to look healthy and, instead, to look at fitness as something you want to do to feel healthy. I want to help you develop a positive relationship to exercise and make it an uplifting and rewarding part of your lifestyle. Total fitness requires consistency and commitment. With the right information, support, and mind-set you *can* incorporate movement into your life as a regular habit.

Now let's look at the three main components of a balanced body fitness program and develop an action plan to get you moving:

- *Cardiovascular training:* burn fat, condition the heart and lungs, boost circulation, and improve mood
- *Strength/resistance training:* build lean muscle mass, boost metabolism, build bone health, prevent injuries, aid in muscular balance, boost performance, and build confidence
- *Flexibility/self-massage training:* ease muscle tension, improve range of motion, decrease stress, and keep muscles happy

Each component is equally important when it comes to beating burnout, but for different reasons. The next three sections are dedicated to explaining each reason thoroughly and giving you guidelines to help you create a personalized balanced body fitness program. I believe movement is medicine that can help you live your best life. Are you ready to be strong, confident, energetic, and unstoppable? Lets start now.

CARDIOVASCULAR FITNESS

The Best Choice

Cardiovascular exercise keeps your heart, lungs, and blood vessels healthy while boosting your metabolism and giving you a good sweat. The best part about aerobic cardio is that there are so many ways to do it. Walking, running, hiking, swimming, biking, taking an aerobics class, dancing, jumping rope—the list goes on. The balanced body breakthrough program lets you personalize your approach to getting your weekly dose of aerobic exercise in a way that you enjoy. Whatever you choose, make it convenient and fun for yourself. If getting your cardio is convenient and enjoyable, you'll stick with it. For example, I love being outside, so running has become one of my favorite ways to get in my cardio. I am also a huge believer in having exercise equipment at home and using workout videos or YouTube channels. It's easy to make time to work out at home: your home is always open, and the weather never prevents you from being active.

When building your cardiovascular fitness, start gradually. There's no rush to go all out in every workout. Take time to condition your heart and lungs until you feel ready to progress and add intensity. If you're new to exercise, start with 20-minute aerobic workouts three times a week (that's the minimum recommended for people who have not exercised regularly), then build to 30 minutes by the third or fourth week. Choose an aerobic activity you know you can stick to. If walking or running is convenient for you, start there. Or sign up for a twice-weekly spin class and join a community with account-ability and support. Or work out at home with a dance aerobics video or an online yoga studio. There are so many options. Think about what you like to do and make it work for you.

As you build your cardiovascular fitness, mix it up and vary your aerobic workouts throughout the week. Change your routine often, varying the intensity, type, or time. This will help you prevent boredom, stay motivated, and continue to see results from your cardio training. Personally, I work out differently depending on my schedule and the weather. I like to spice up my routine by trying different group fitness classes or new running trails. Here are a few great ways to change up your workouts.

Intensity

Varying the intensity of your aerobic workouts will allow you to be more consistent and avoid injury. Think about it: if you do too many *high-intensity* workouts, you'll burn out fast. If you do too many *low-intensity* workouts you'll plateau and won't see continued results. Vary your weekly workouts from low, to medium, to high.

- *Low-intensity cardio training*—for example, walking, hiking, and slow cycling—can be done practically every day (even several times a day) for longer amounts of time than high-intensity training. This type of training is very easy for your body to recover from, regardless of your body type and your goals. It can help you burn calories for fat loss and help you build lifestyle fitness.

- *Moderate-intensity cardio training*—for example, jogging, swimming, stair climbing, cross-country skiing, cycling, ice skating, aerobics, step aerobics, and dancing—will need to be done a little less frequently. This type of training requires more energy to do and to recover from.
- *High-intensity training*—for example, activities like sprinting, circuit workouts, and interval training—is the toughest of the three but can actually bring you the fastest results. High-intensity training is extremely effective for fat loss as it not only causes you to burn a lot of calories during the activity, but it also raises your metabolism for a long time after the activity is done. This type of hard training should be done less frequently than the more moderate forms of cardio as it is much harder for your body to recover.

Please don't allow yourself to become frustrated by sticking to only one intensity level for your workouts. I alternate high-impact aerobics or hard running days with swimming and cycling. This allows me to continue consistent workouts without getting injured or bored, or hitting a plateau.

Type

I hate it when I hear people say that they are running to get a workout but hate running. That's crazy. If you hate running, don't run! There are so many options to try when it comes to getting your cardio that there is no reason to torture yourself with something you don't like. Anything you don't enjoy will result in mediocre efforts and mediocre results. Find forms of cardio workouts that you enjoy, and you won't feel like you're working. Make it fun and you'll stick with it in the long run.

Here's a list of great cardio activities to help you figure out what you like to do: running, walking, swimming, aerobics, water aerobics, step aerobics, jump rope, boxing, rowing, cycling, indoor cycling, treadmill intervals, dancing, elliptical machine, stair climbing, hiking, rowing, tennis, basketball, and soccer.

Variety

You can also add variety in the frequency of your cardio workouts. Maybe one week you choose to do three running workouts and the next you choose to do two aerobics classes and one swim. This will keep your body guessing, and the results will keep happening.

One of my personal favorite ways to spice up my cardio is to alternate between steady-state aerobics and interval training workouts. *Steady state* means staying in an aerobic state for a set period of time. *Interval training* means alternating between high and low intensity throughout the duration of your workout. This gives you many options for cardio. You can alternate going on a steady-state walk or jog with an interval-based cycling or aerobic class. Interval training has been shown to be more effective for seeing results than steady-state aerobic training. However, it's important to build your aerobic fitness too, and if you do interval training for all your workouts you'll burn out! Aim to alternate interval-based workouts with steady-state aerobic workouts. This will allow you to continue to see results and benefit from your cardiovascular training.

Whatever you do, don't get stuck in a rut. Your body and mind love when you mix it up. These guidelines should help give you an idea of different modes, intensities, and types of cardio to help you continue to craft a plan custom fit for you.

Take these recommendations simply as advice—not as rules written in stone—and feel free to experiment. Your cardio schedule will continue to change as you progress and adjust your fitness goals. Don't be afraid to try something new. Your exercise options are in no way limited to what you learned in high school gym, and there is a fitness fit out there for everyone!

Now you know some ways to make your cardio fun, effective, and part of your balanced life. Change your workout routine every two to four weeks to avoid plateaus, injuries, and burnout. Start with at least 30 minutes of cardio exercise three times a week and go from there. That's 90 minutes of movement—and you can do it. Workouts can sometimes be difficult, but they're not a chore. Make them an adventure, and make them fun. Do that, and you'll smile all the way to the finish line—and beyond.

STRENGTH TRAINING FOR A POWERFUL LIFE

Consistent and smart strength training played a powerful role for me in overcoming burnout and living a balanced life. While movement was always a part of my world, I didn't learn how to have a balanced strength-training program until 2011. Before that, the only "strength" I did was holding a plank or doing a group fitness class with eight-pound weights. I didn't have a consistent strength routine. My workouts involved repetitive movements and I developed muscular imbalances that caused injury, followed by more burnout. I kept trying to fix myself with more of the same bad exercise habits—too much endurance training, too much stretching, no smart strength training—and I kept getting the same results: more injuries and more burnout. That's a terrible cycle to be in. Injuries cause burnout, which in turn cause depression, low self-esteem, and sadness. The only way to get out of the cycle is to stop the madness. Stop doing what's *not* working, and develop a plan that *will* work.

To really take care of my body, I needed to make a change, and what my body needed more of was strength. Because I didn't really know where to start, I hired a coach to help me build a plan from the ground up. She put together a program custom-fit to my needs that helped me build strength and body symmetry. My plan involved getting on the weight room floor and reuniting with my hips, glutes, hamstrings, and core. I needed to restore the power in my muscles and stabilize my joints. I did squats. I deadlifted. I swung kettlebells. I did rows. The strength training healed my stress-related injuries and allowed me to recover from burnout. More important, it enabled me to become a new version of myself: a stronger, more confident, injury-proof woman.

Today, strength training is a healthy habit I can't live without. Since it became a consistent part of my life, I haven't had an injury and am able to do all the activities I love with ease, gratitude, and joy. Many people are scared of strength training or find it intimidating. I want to encourage you to start now, learn the ropes, and give yourself the gift of strength.

Strength training is an essential component to the balanced body exercise program. The American College of Sports Medicine (ACSM) recommends a minimum of two strength sessions per week to develop and maintain strong muscles.

Consistent strength training for a minimum of 20 minutes twice per week will allow you to achieve the following benefits.

Get the body you want.

Lean, toned muscles and more definition are what you want, so how do you get more toned? Light weights and lots of reps, right? At least that's what we've been told to believe. However, training to "get toned" with lots of reps and light weights will not provide the same benefits as lifting properly with heavy weights. Getting toned requires two things to happen:

- Ridding the body of excess fat
- Increasing the size of muscle cells to provide shape

Toning is all about building muscle. For some, it requires the additional removal of any fat covering up the muscle, but it is muscle itself that gives you sleek, sculpted curves once you lose excess body fat. So how do you lose body fat and increase lean muscle concurrently? Combine a healthy amount of cardio/aerobic exercise—high-intensity interval training (HIIT), sprint-type workouts, and plyometrics (jump training)—with one to three weight workouts a week with weights that are just the right challenge for you (heavyish weight with proper form).

Strengthen bones and muscles.

Lifting weights builds muscles, and it makes for stronger bones. Did you know an average woman can lose up to 1 percent of bone mineral density every year? For men, it is not quite as much, but it adds up! After the age of twenty-five, we lose more than one half pound of muscle every year without a regular strength-training regimen. Add strength training and work to prevent osteoporosis. When you strength train, the act of moving your bones through muscle action increases their density. Your skeletal system becomes stronger in response to the demands that strength exercise places on your body. As you age, increased bone density will reduce the risk of fractures and chronic disease. According to the American College of Sports Medicine (ACSM), you can significantly reduce your risk of developing osteoporosis by engaging in regular weight training workouts.

Burn more calories.

We tend to think of cardiovascular exercise as the calorie burner necessary for losing weight. However, it's better to lose inches and gain muscle than to just simply lose pounds. Muscle, unlike fat, is metabolically active. Cardio burns calories during the workout. Strength training burns calories both during and after the workout. It was reported in the *Journal of Strength and Conditioning Research* that women who completed an hour-long strength-training workout burned an average of 100 more calories in the 24 hours afterward than they did when they hadn't lifted weights. Replace 10 pounds of fat with 10 pounds of lean muscle, and you can burn an additional 25 to 50 calories a day without even trying. This "afterburn" effect is the metabolism boost needed to maintain a healthy weight over time and maximize your calorie burn.

Lose more fat.

In addition to burning more calories, resistance training may help your body to burn more fat overall. Score! In one study of more than 700 women, lifting weights for just 25 minutes three times per week led to the gain of nearly two pounds of muscle and the loss of four pounds of fat. If you're familiar with how physiques work, then you know that is a radical change in appearance! Now, picking up heavy things burns a respectable amount of calories on its own. No doubt about that. But that's not why lifting weights is so effective for burning fat. Rather, when you lift something heavy, you're setting your body up for metabolic reactions that allow you to utilize nutrients better and continue burning calories for up to 36 hours after your workout. The basal metabolic rate (BMR) controls how many calories your body burns while you rest. As you gain more muscle, you increase your BMR, along with how much you can eat and still stay lean. The more lean muscle on your body, the less body fat you will store, and the harder it will be to gain weight.

It is important to remember that losing fat may cause noticeable changes in your body (e.g. decrease in size, increase in tone) when looking in the mirror, but the number on the scales may not change. This is because resistance training can increase the amount of lean muscle you have, which is heavier but takes up less space than fat. Simply put, if fat goes down but muscle goes up, your weight could essentially stay the same. I'm talking about the difference between weight loss and fat loss and why you should focus on fitness, not skinniness, for long-term health. Check out the photo below to remind you that lean muscle may weigh more but takes up less space than fat.

Have better posture.
Stronger bones will improve your posture and how you carry yourself. Weight training can ensure that the muscles between the shoulder blades, lower back, and abdomen stay strong, which reduces the likelihood of developing muscular imbalances that can lead to poor posture. Better posture will enhance your overall appearance and reduce your chances of suffering from back pain or injury.

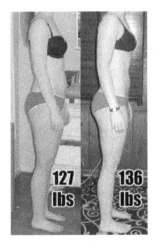

Ease joint pain and prevent injuries.

Muscles function as shock absorbers and serve as important balancing agents throughout the body. Well-conditioned muscles help to lessen the repetitive landing force in weight-bearing activities such as running or basketball. Also, well-balanced muscles reduce the risk of injuries that result from muscular imbalances. (Super strong quads and weak hamstrings?! Not with smart strength training.) Build a foundation of strength, and you'll be less likely to run into injury from sports or daily activities. Stronger muscles hold your joints in position better, so you won't need to worry about, for example, your knee pain flaring up during your next run.

Impress yourself with progress.

The amazing thing about resistance training and lifting weights in general is that you are able to see how far you've come. For example, you may have started weighted lunges with 10-pound dumbbells, barely making it through your set, and weeks later you can easily do them with 20-pound dumbbells. I love weight training because you can see and feel that you have improved, and that is very satisfying. Such progress can encourage you to keep going and continue to improve.

Reduce your risk of heart disease and diabetes.

As we age, we lose muscle mass, which makes us weaker and more prone to weight gain. Resistance training can help slow down age-related muscle loss, which means that not only will you look better, but you also are protecting your health. During exercise, muscle tissue helps to remove additional glucose and triglycerides from your bloodstream, which can help to reduce your risk of type 2 diabetes and heart disease. There is also evidence suggesting that resistance training can help with high blood pressure.

Kick ass.

Yes, you heard right! When you are stronger, fitter, and have more endurance, you will automatically become better at other movement-based activities that you attempt—like lifting your suitcase into the overhead bin on the airplane, arm wrestling your brother, carrying all six grocery bags at once, lifting (and keeping up with) your kids, moving boxes and furniture in your house, opening a pickle jar, and on and on. . . .

Maximize your gym time.

Cardio sessions can sometimes take up a good portion of an hour, which can be tricky to squeeze in before work or between commitments. Fortunately, with resistance training, you don't need to spend hours at the gym. All you need is a 20- to 60-minute lifting session about three times a week to start seeing great results in as little as two weeks. However, I like to reinforce this efficiency mind-set with all of my trainees: Get In. Work Hard. Get Out. You'll have more time to spend with your favorite people and to do your favorite things.

Build a nice butt.

Want a nice booty? The gluteus maximus is one of the strongest muscles in your body. The shape of your glutes are influenced by muscular development. When it comes to building size in your glutes, there is no substitute for a deep, heavy squat. This will also help rid you of cellulite, while "firming" and "toning" your legs in the process. You'll also strengthen your lower back and help prevent back injuries that are all too common as we age.

Change your body shape.

You may think your genes determine how you look. That's not necessarily true. Weight training can slim you down, create new curves, and help avoid the "middle-age spread." Even dropping just 3 percent of your body fat could translate into a total loss of 3 inches off your hips and thighs.

Boost your flexibility.

Researchers from the University of North Dakota pitted static stretches against strength-training exercises and found that full-range resistance training workouts can improve flexibility just as well as your typical static stretching regimen. That means exercises like squats and lunges can boost your flexibility in addition to your strength. The key term here is *full range*. If you can't complete the full motion—going all the way up and all the way down—with a given weight, you may need to use a lighter dumbbell and work up to it.

Get more energy.

Exercise produces endorphins (natural opiates produced by the brain). They make you happy, you feel great, and you have more energy! Have you ever had a workout during which you were really in the moment—putting your mind into the muscle or movements at hand, giving 100 percent effort? How did you feel afterward? Perhaps, initially, you felt a bit tired, but chances are that you left the workout with a new spring in your step—renewed energy. Lifting heavy weights challenges you in new ways, leaving you with newfound energy you got from that workout. Strength training has also been shown to help you sleep better (since your muscles are craving recovery, rest, and repair post-workout)—and better sleep equals more energy in the long run.

Boost your body image.

Lifting weights can help shift the focus of your body image from size to ability. In other words, instead of focusing on your weight or the size of your waist, you'll begin to better appreciate your body for its strength and what it can do. When we focus on actual fitness instead of body size, more muscle can mean more ease in moving our bodies, promoting better relationships with our bodies and with exercise.

Gain confidence.

You know it: exercise boosts the ego—it helps you feel great in your own skin. The foundation of building inner confidence (and self-belief) lies in setting goals that may seem beyond your capabilities and working toward them (consistently and with commitment) until you achieve them. And there's something about strength training that makes you feel, well . . . strong. And that feeling of inner strength—that your muscles are growing, you're developing definition, and you're boosting your metabolism—works as a powerful confidence-booster.

At this point you're probably thinking that everything sounds amazing but have this voice in your head telling you that you're going to get big or bulky. I hear this far too often. It's simply a misbelief that is holding you back from seeing results quickly. Get it out of your head right this second; you will *not* look like a bodybuilder if you add regular weight training to your workout routine. In fact you may finally achieve that lean, toned body you are killing yourself over with all that cardio. How do you know it won't work if you haven't really tried it? It's worth a shot. Get ready to be impressed with your body and your results.

If you are really still worried about gaining size and becoming the next Incredible Hulk, consider this: bodybuilders are doing everything in their power to build muscle, and they are still struggling. It's very difficult to see massive muscle gains, unless, of course, you're training like a monster, consuming a massive amount of calories, and injecting yourself with synthetic hormones. When you follow a strength-training program customized to fit your body's needs and goals, you'll see the results you want—not the extra bulk.

Ready to pump some iron? Here are a few questions and answers to help you get started on the road toward strength success.

How often should I strength train?

I recommend you strength train, at a minimum, at least twice a week. This number has been shown to provide many of the health benefits of resistance training. In a perfect world, three or four times per week is ideal. I like to do heavy, total-body strength workouts in the weight room two times a week and one or two days of lighter/endurance strength training, such as Pilates, group fitness weight-training classes, or body-weight exercises. You can strength train on the same days you do your aerobic training if your week is too busy for separate 30-minute workouts.

How much weight should I use?

Choose the heaviest weight that allows you to complete all the set repetitions in each exercise with good form. In other words, the lower the number of repetitions, the heavier the weight you should use and vice versa. Just make sure the weight allows you to perform the exercise properly—lifting less weight with good form is better than lifting more weight sloppily. If you are doing body-weight exercises (using your body weight as resistance), the same principal applies: perform as many reps as you can in each set with good form.

How do you figure out the right amount to lift?

The answer is trial and error. You have to make an educated guess and experiment. The key is to start lifting. If you choose a weight that's too light or too heavy, adjust it in your next set. The goal is to complete all the repetitions in each set with good form while challenging your muscles to work as hard as they can. Using the "start to struggle" approach will help you do this: work hard; when you start to struggle, you've completed the set. This is also a good strategy to use for body-weight exercises such as push-ups, pull-ups, and hip raises.

How many repetitions should I do?

How many reps you choose to do depends on the specific exercise and your training goals. Start by trying to complete 8 to 15 repetitions of each exercise. In the beginning, if you can only do 5 repetitions with good form, then 5 is fine. Gradually begin to increase the number as the exercise gets easier. If you can accomplish 20 or more, it's time to add more weight. If you want to build more muscle and strength, add more weight and decrease the repetitions to between 5 and 10. What is most important is that you listen to your body. Do what you can, and increase from there. Most important to remember is that this is *your* program. Make it start where you are and build from there.

How many sets of an exercise should I do?

Start with 2 or 3 sets of an exercise. For example, if you are doing 3 sets of 10 reps of a chest press, that's 30 chest presses total. As you develop your strength, you can play around with a variety of sets and reps. That's the fun part!

How many exercises should I do per muscle group?

Start with one exercise per muscle group to keep it simple. The muscle groups are butt, hamstrings, quads, chest, back, biceps, triceps, shoulders, and abdominals. The American Council on Exercise website is a fabulous resource for learning proper form and great strength-training moves.

Do I need equipment or gym access in order to start strength training?

You don't. You can begin a strength-training program with body-weight exercises: push-ups, squats, lunges, bridges, planks, and more. There's an endless list of no-equipment-needed movements you can do to build strength. However, in order to continue to progress and see positive results, you will eventually want to consider adding resistance. Whether you purchase weights to use at home, register for a strength-training class, or join a gym, having access to weight-training equipment will allow you to have the ability to progress with your strength training.

How do I learn proper form?

When developing your personal weight-training routine, it's best to start by consulting with a personal trainer or coach to establish a program that suits your specific needs and abilities. If you're not familiar with the basic principles of strength training, a fitness professional can give you the guidance you need to start strong. Working with a trainer to establish a foundation of strength-training knowledge and good form can get you started with safe and effective program. As always, if you have any medical conditions, injuries, or illnesses, be sure to check with your doctor before you start lifting weights.

When should I start?

It's never too late to start. Strength training can help you take your body to the next level, while also having a number of positive effects on your overall health. Don't be afraid to lift weights! Just keep in mind that resistance training is not the only solution to achieving your health and fitness goals. Instead, focus on creating a balanced exercise program, consisting of strength training and cardio training, while also planning time for reha-bilitation and rest.

I believe in strength training because I have seen it change my body, boost my performance, and give me the power to beat burnout. I also believe you deserve a chance to discover your own strength. So here's to you living without limits.

FLEXIBILITY TRAINING AND SELF-MASSAGE

Chronic stress causes the body to malfunction. When you are mentally or physically burned out, your body knows it. You suffer from random aches and pains. You randomly pull mus-cles or tweak something. Addressing your stress is the first step to better health. Moving your body on a daily basis is part of that. That's why regular stretching and self-massage are part of the balanced body program. They will reset and recharge you to allow you to achieve your optimal state of well-being and performance. Regular self-massage and flexibility training will untangle knots of tension and give you the tools to elimi-nate pain and move past stress-related injuries. It also will help keep your joints mobile so that your body lasts longer and is pain free for decades.

If you sit most of the day and are under a lot of stress, your body is tight and hungry for some relief. Self-massage and flex-ibility training provide the best way to tame that tension. Your goal is a minimum of 5 to 10 minutes of flexibility or self-mas-sage exercises daily. You can choose to do them at the end of a workout, throughout your day, or even before bed. What matters most is that you make time to do it. A few minutes go a long way and will help reduce muscle soreness, limber your joints, improve range of motion, release tension, and beat stress-related injuries. I'm going to teach you how easy it is to fit in simple stretches and self-massage throughout your day. Soon it will be a healthy habit, like brushing your teeth. You'll feel so much better from just a few minutes of moving and deep breathing. Start with a daily stretch following any YouTube "Quick, Effective Stretching Videos" and notice how you feel.

Now let's get foam-rolling. I believe self-massage is a powerful tool to beating burnout and feeling good. The only thing you need to start a self-massage routine is the right equipment.

Not all gyms provide foam rollers, and it will be worth your while to purchase your own tools for home use. Most foam-rolling devices cost between $10 and $40 and are much more affordable than hiring your own massage therapist. Having self-massage tools at home will make it easy to fit in 5 to 10 minutes of daily self-massage. You might find that it becomes a habit you look forward to every day because it feels so good. When it comes to which foam-rolling tools to purchase, you have several different options. Here are my favorites:

- High-density foam roller: A compact, high-density roller is designed to maintain its shape. It is the most common self-massage tool you will find at gyms and fitness centers.
- The grid: This travel-ready roller with a foam grid is designed for trigger-point release.
- Yoga Tune Up balls: The Yoga Tune Up therapy balls measure about 2½ inches in diameter each and are made of a special rubber that grips skin, grabs at multiple layers of muscles, and rubs out adhesions and tension, providing a deep tissue massage. These are great for traveling and taking to work for self-massage as they pack well in a suitcase or purse.

- Golf ball: Perfect for getting all the tiny spots in your feet, a golf ball can aid in healing plantar fasciitis and other not-so-fun foot problems.
- Rolling pin: I use a standard kitchen rolling pin as an inexpensive, on-the-go massage tool. It's easy to travel with and can be useful in working out the kinks in my calves, quads, and iliotibial (IT) band.

Disclaimer: Always check with your doctor before using a foam roller for myofascial release. Also, foam-rolling a tight muscle may cause discomfort, which usually means the area needs attention. Perform foam roller sessions when your muscles are warm or after a workout. Each time you use your foam roller makes the next time a little bit easier. Just don't forget to breathe.

Foam-roll like a pro. Here's how:

- You can choose to foam-roll before a workout to loosen up, after a workout to cool down, or any time of day to release tension from the body.
- Position the roller under the soft tissue area you want to release or loosen.
- Place your body part on the roller and apply pressure. Stay in place or gently roll your body weight back and forth across the roller while targeting the affected muscle.
- Move slowly, and take deep breaths.
- If you find a particularly painful area (trigger point), hold that position until the area softens.
- Focus on areas that are tight or have reduced range of motion.
- Roll over each area a few times until you feel it relax. Expect some discomfort. It may feel very tender at first.

- Stay on soft tissue and avoid rolling directly over bones or joints.
- Keep your first few foam roller sessions short. Aim to foam-roll an area for a minimum of 2 minutes to create change in the tissues.
- Rest a day between sessions when you start.

I carry my Yoga Tune Up balls with me everywhere I go. I use them in the car on my lower back while driving or fit in a neck massage in the office between meetings. Having them on hand makes it easy to fit a quick massage into small windows of time throughout the day. Search on YouTube for foam-rolling videos for more ideas on how to use these tools for self care.

I believe 5 to 10 minutes of flexibility and self-massage training every day insure against the likelihood of injury and the aches and pains that result from stored tension in the muscles. If this sounds impossible, try to stretch for at least 2 minutes at the end of your workouts. You can also squeeze in a few quick stretches in line at the grocery store, before bed, or even while brushing your teeth. Opportunities to stretch, breathe, roll, release, and de-stress exist everywhere if you look for them. Which leads us into the next section: how to fit in more movement throughout your day.

ACTIVE LIVING: HOW TO LIVE FIT

Living a more active life starts with a mind-set shift. You have to be willing to drop the all-or-nothing mind-set and look for ways to get moving every chance you get. Exercise is not limited to your workouts. Don't aim only to be active for 30 minutes three times a week—aim to integrate more activity into your daily life. Doing so will help keep you mobile, happy, and fit. You'll be up for anything—a mover who can handle life's challenges with ease. Here are my suggestions for making more movement happen and living a fit lifestyle that fuels everything you do with health:

- Take 5 minutes in the morning to stretch, breathe, and move your body.
- If you start your day in a stressful way, you'll probably feel stressed for the rest of the day. Do 5 minutes of movement in the morning to start your day with energy. Side bends, squats, downward dog—whatever feels good to you. Beginning the day in this way will make you more relaxed and give you a strong start.
- Walk as much as possible. Get some steps when you can, wherever you can! You might be busy and think that every minute is valuable time to put into your work, but some extra minutes of walking might be a better way to spend some time. If you live close to where you're going, it's better to walk than to use your car or public transportation. Not only will the exercise be good for you, but you also will get some essential fresh air and daylight. If you have to commute and use public transportation, get off one or two stops early; if you drive to work, park your car farther away than usual. Get creative and find ways to take extra steps. Even a few minutes of movement will help you feel more focused and relaxed.
- Mix socializing with exercising. Do you normally spend time with family or friends by going to dinner, watching sports on TV, or going to movies? Make your social time more active by planning events that get all of you moving. Go for a family hike on a beautiful Saturday morning, play a game of tag football with your buddies during halftime, or make a date for a run with your significant other or best

friend. Personally, I love scheduling "healthy hour" dates to enjoy a walk or workout with my friends. I believe you can build strong relationships through movement and bond over the effort, endorphins, and sense of accomplishment. There are so many options for including more activity in your social life. Next time someone wants to plan a get-to-gether, suggest something that involves exercise.

• When you are too busy for a workout, find 5 minutes to move somewhere in your day. Do it at the office, right when you get home, or even while waiting for the bus. Any time is better than no time when it comes to moving for energy and self-care.

• Make working out accessible. Work out outside or at home. Sometimes getting to the gym simply isn't an option, but that doesn't have to stop you from getting exercise.

Working Out at Home

The following are a few great resources to help you work out wherever your life finds you—no equipment required!

Working Out with Free Videos
10 Best YouTube Channels for Free Fitness Videos, available at Mashable.com.

Online Fitness/Yoga Studios
Yogaglo and Fitnessglo. Great fitness classes at all different levels and lengths for a small monthly fee. Workout anywhere, anytime.

Best Home Workout Smartphone Apps

The following apps are perfect workout companions and will keep you motivated and well equipped at home:

- Nike Training Club. Nike's personal training app gives you access to a personal trainer anytime, anywhere. The app offers more than 85 custom-built workouts with detailed instructions and audio commentary. It also tracks the details and history of all your workouts. (Free; iOS and Android)
- Sworkit. Tell Sworkit the type of workout you're looking for (strength, cardio, yoga, or stretching) and the amount of time you've got (anywhere from five minutes to an hour), and the app delivers the moves to follow during your sweat session. If you opt for premium ($4.99 per month), the app lets you get even more personalized, by setting the number of reps and the areas of the body you want to focus on. (Free with optional in-app purchases; iOS and Android)
- Daily Burn. Stream a workout directly to your phone or computer anytime with the DailyBurn app. Access a carefully curated library of live workouts and professional-quality fitness videos. A panel of expert trainers (specializing in different areas of fitness) keep you on your toes through each exercise session. From yoga to cardio kickboxing to dancing to kettlebells, this app has a workout video to suit any fitness preference and goal. Free for 30 days; online subscription, $12.95 monthly. (iOS and Android)
- Couch to 5K. If you've wanted to try running but never known where to start, Couch to 5K should be the next app you download. The free eight-week program gives users three workouts per week that get you ready for your local Turkey Trot or Fourth of July road race. (Free; iOS and Android)

- Freeletics. Looking for bodyweight workouts? Freeletics has more than 900 that last anywhere from 10 to 30 minutes. Whether you choose to work out in the kitchen, on the subway, or in your office, you can rely on Freeletics to deliver a great workout for your fitness level. (Free; iOS and Android)
- Daily Yoga. Never be bored by yoga again. More than 50 classes shot in HD video are just a few taps away. Each sequence has a specific focus, from increasing flexibility to strengthening your core. Plus, there's a library with detailed videos of more than 500 poses. (Free with optional in-app purchases; iOS and Android)
- ExerciseTV. Every day, you'll get a 10- to 40-minute workout video ranging from aerobics to yoga from ExerciseTV. A light hand weight is the only piece of equipment you might need, but you can always use a filled water bottle. (Free; iOS and Android)
- Fitbit. Track your progress, connect with your friends, join challenges, and stay motivated with this easy to use app from Fitbit. (Free; iOS and Android)
- FitStar Personal Trainer. You no longer have to cough up the big bucks for a personal trainer to get workouts tailored directly for you. FitStar personal trainer assesses your needs and fitness level by asking you a simple set of questions at the end of every workout. That way every workout is challenging but doesn't crush you. The program's offerings are a good fit for everyone from beginners to fitness fanatics—after all, it was created by former NFL star Tony Gonzalez. (Free; iOS)

Staying Active at the Office

Putting in too much time in the office chair is dangerous. But these days too many of us are pulling crazy hours at work and our health is suffering for it. Spending too much time sitting has been linked to a higher risk of heart attack, stroke, metabolic syndrome, and earlier death, and unfortunately even the most dedicated exercise regimens won't undo all the damage, not to mention the rising increase of desk job–related injuries like carpal tunnel, tennis elbow, frozen shoulder, wrist strain, neck and shoulder pain, sciatica, hip pain, and lower back pain.

I believe we are built to move. It's stress and *not* moving that are the hardest on our bodies and health long term. Have you ever had an achy back from a long day of sitting? Or a serious headache from too much time staring at a computer screen? You are not alone. Pretty much 99 percent of my corporate clients struggle with pain from too much time at a desk and dealing with work-related stress. Lucky for you the solution is simple and doesn't require a ton of time. I am here because I want to help you feel better. And I promise you: simply taking the time to move more in the office will dramatically improve how your body feels.

If you work at a desk or spend a lot of time on tech, I have some life hacks you can use to prevent the dangerous side effects of sitting and stress. Here are my secrets to success. Are you ready to feel better yet?

Sitting Hurts. How To Get Fit and Get Fixed Fast.

- Move every hour. Aim to get up and out of your seat at least every hour. Even if you just swing your arms or take a deep breath, you'll feel more alert.

- Fit in stretching and strength exercises intermittently throughout your day. Aim to stretch the hip flexors, shoulders, lower back, hips, and chest. Aim to engage the upper back, core, and glutes.
- Walk as much as possible: hand-deliver reports or discuss an issue in person instead of via e-mail. Researchers find that adding 2 minutes of light exercise to each hour of your day lowers your risk of dying prematurely by 33 percent. Get your heart pumping, blood flowing, give your energy a boost, and rev your metabolism every hour with 2 minutes of walking or movement every hour.
- Wear comfortable shoes to work (or even walk to and from work) if you can. Keep a pair of dress shoes with you or in the office, and put them on only when necessary.
- Fill your water bottle. Drink it and replenish it often. (This might result in a few extra trips to the bathroom, but that gives you more opportunity to move!) Stand up and take the long way to the water cooler.
- Sit on an exercise ball instead of a chair. This will strengthen your abs and back, and you'll work on your posture without even trying.
- Use the restroom on another floor and take the stairs.
- Use an activity tracker to keep track of how many steps you take. Working with a step counter or a more sophisticated activity tracker can tell you exactly how active you are during your work hours. This may provide you good insight as to the importance of fitness during your hectic workday. I'm addicted to my Fitbit. Aim for 6,000 to 10,000 steps each day.
- Eat your lunch away from your desk. Walk to a lunch place or go to a nearby park. Enjoy a longer route back to the office when you're done.
- Have walking meetings. Invite colleagues to join you on a walking meeting or take your calls on a headset so you

can move around while you talk. Researchers at Stanford University found that the creative output of people increases by an average of 60 percent when they are walking. Indoor walks were found to be just as effective for boosting creativity as outdoor walks. Get "sweatworking" and find a way to incorporate movement into your meetings.

- A good goal is small exercises, like stretches every 30 to 40 minutes, and large exercises, like walking around the office or taking the stairs every 90 minutes. Never go 2 hours without moving! You can do it!

Staying Active While Traveling

Travel can be exhausting and stressful, which makes exercise an important part of maintaining your health when you are away from home. Although travel schedules, irregular mealtimes, unfamiliar sleeping arrangements and other stressors can take their toll, you can do a number of things to make travel less draining. Start by focusing on ways to get healthy exercise on any trip you take. You may not have time to fit in a long workout on the road, but even short bouts of exercise and stretching will prove beneficial.

- A successful trip begins before you leave home. *Plan for success* by researching your destination.
  Learn about the area as well as your intended accommodations. Find out about the fitness amenities at your hotel, and if possible book one that offers a well-equipped gym or in-room yoga or fitness videos and fitness sessions for guests. You can use Google or Yelp to locate fitness facilities, running trails, yoga classes, and other wellness services.
- If you fly, *pay attention to opportunities for exercise.*

You can walk and stretch at any airport, and some airports offer walking tracks or Zen rooms for travelers. During your flight, be sure to do some stretches and in-flight exercise. This will help you avoid cramping, stiffness, and other discomforts frequently associated with travel.

- When you arrive at your destination, take time to orient yourself to your surroundings before dashing off to meetings or other activities. Locate the amenities at your hotel, including the fitness center. In your room, familiarize yourself with the space and do a few yoga poses or simple breathing exercises to center yourself.
- *Keep your expectations realistic, and make little bits of time count.*

  Few trips will accommodate your regular exercise routine, and chances are that you won't have time to work out for an hour or so each day. You will, however, have several opportunities to get some movement. Take the stairs instead of an elevator whenever possible. Get a little exercise by walking to meetings or meals instead of riding or driving.
- *Never minimize any exercise opportunities you get while traveling.*

  Small windows of time can turn into powerful opportunities for health and fitness. When you take advantage of them, your travel will be considerably less stressful. You'll return home feeling more energized and also find it easier to return to your usual exercise routine after the trip.

Need some exercise ideas to get you going? Here are my favorite no-equipment-needed moves that you can do anywhere. Put them together in a sequence, or choose to do one for more energy at some point in your day. A little movement goes a long way, and one exercise is always better than zero!

Core Exercises

Plank

Lie face-down on the floor with your legs together, forearms close to the torso, and toes perpendicular to the floor as if you're going to do a push up. Lift your body using your abdominal muscles and

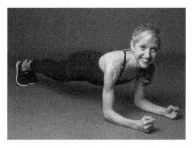

your arms, until it's in a straight line from head to toe, and the only body parts touching the floor are your toes and your forearms. Hold this position for as long as you can, working up to three minutes at a time. A good starting goal is 2-3 sets of 30-60 seconds.

Single leg drop

Lie on the floor with the legs extended up in the air above your hips. Place the hands underneath your hips or at your sides. Lower one leg down toward the floor and bring leg back up to meet the other. Repeat with single legs or take both legs down at the same time. Try 2-3 sets of 12-20 reps.

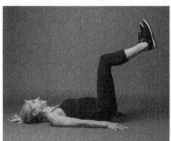
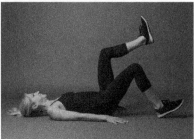

Push-Up to Side Plank

Combine push-up and plank and get the best bang for your buck! Starting in plank, perform one push-up. After coming back up into a starting push-up position, rotate your body to the right and extend the right hand overhead, forming a side plank with arms in a T position. Return to the starting position, do a normal push-up, then rotate to the left.

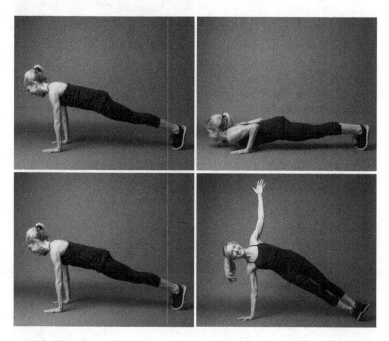

Bicycle

Lie down with knees bent and hands behind the head. With the knees in toward the chest, bring the right elbow toward the left knee as the right leg straightens. Continue alternating sides. Go slowly, focus on form, and aim to keep the shoulders off the ground with the elbows open.

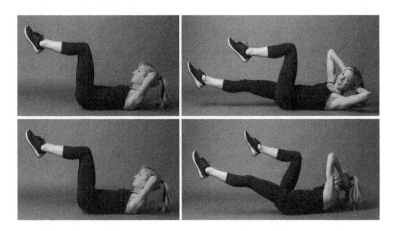

Crunch

Form is key when it comes to this exercise standby. Lie on your back with the knees bent and feet flat on the floor. With hands behind the head, place the chin down slightly and peel the head and shoulders off the mat while engaging the core. Continue curling up until the upper back is off the mat. Hold briefly, then lower the torso back toward the mat slowly.

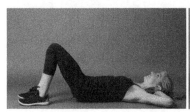 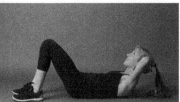

Windshield Wipers

This move helps you target the oblique muscles. Lying on your back with your knees bent and core tight, let the knees fall gradually to the left. You should feel a stretch in your lower back, but use your core to control the legs. Hold for five seconds, return to center, and repeat on the right side.

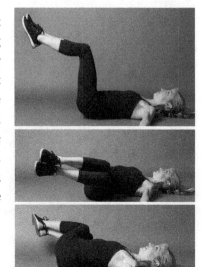

Hip Bridge

Lie on your back with the knees bent and feet hip-width apart. Place arms at your side and lift up the spine and hips. Slowly bring the hips back down, then lift back up. Try to do 10-20 reps or try 10 reps of single leg hip bridge with one leg in the air.

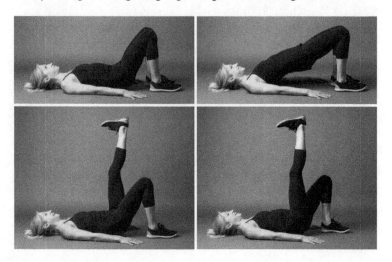

Single Leg Stretch

Lie on your back with knees in a tabletop position. Lift your head and shoulders off the ground, bring one knee in toward your nose and extend other leg straight out. Wrap your arms around bent knee. Switch legs and alternate for 10-20 reps. Keep your head on the floor, if needed, for your neck.

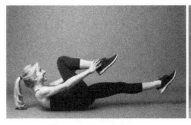 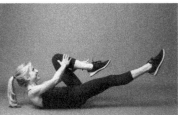

Single Straight Leg Stretch

Lie on your back with knees in a tabletop position. Lift your head and shoulders off the ground, and extend one leg straight in the air and the other leg straight out a few inches off the floor. Wrap your arms around the straight leg in the air. Lift your shoulders off the floor to feel your core and keep your neck in neutral. Feel a nice stretch in your hamstrings as you scissor switch the legs for 10-20 reps. Keep your head on the floor if needed for your neck.

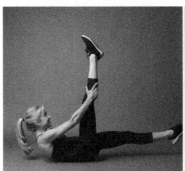 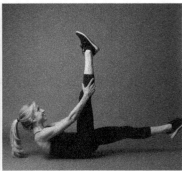

Double Leg Stretch

Two legs is twice the fun. Lie on your back with knees in a tabletop position. Lift your head and shoulders off the ground, bring both knees in toward your nose and wrap your arms around your knees. Extend both legs out at the same time, reaching the arms beyond the head. Scoop your arms back around as you bring the knees back in towards your nose and repeat. Try 10-20 reps. Keep your head on the floor, if needed, for your neck.

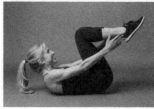 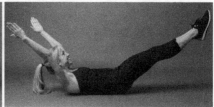

Side Plank

Lift your body on the side with one elbow and foot (or knee as shown). Make sure your hips are lifted and your core is engaged. Hold this position for 30-60 seconds and then repeat on the second side. Try different variations for challenge.

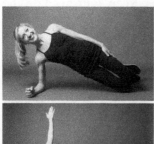 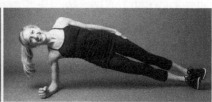

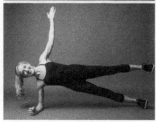

Sprinter Sit-Up

Lie on your back with your legs straight and arms by your side—elbows bent at a 90-degree angle. Now sit up, bringing your left knee toward the right elbow. Lower your body and repeat on the other side.

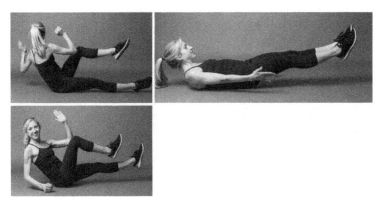

Russian Twist

Sit on the floor with knees bent and feet together, lifted a few inches off the floor. With your back at a 45-degree angle from the ground, move the arms from one side to another in a twisting motion. Here, slow and steady wins the race: the slower the twist, the deeper the burn.

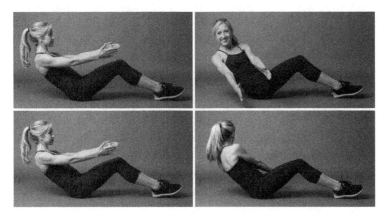

Lower Body Exercises

Wall Sit

Place your back against a wall. Slide down the wall until your thighs are parallel to the ground. Make sure your knees are directly above your ankles and keep your back straight. Hold for 30-60 seconds. Need more of a challenge? Add bicep curls or hold your arms out straight.

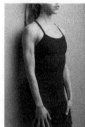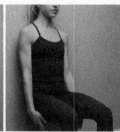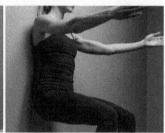

Lunge

Stand with hands on hips and feet hip-width apart. Step your right leg backward and lower your body until your right knee is close to or touching the floor and bent at least 90 degrees. Return to the starting position and repeat with left leg. Try stepping forward into the lunge for a different variation. Make sure your knees are behind your toes when you lunge. Work on your posture, keeping your upper body tall with shoulders back and chest open.

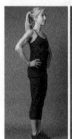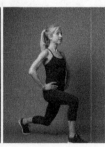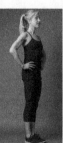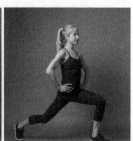

Clock Lunge

Complete a traditional forward lunge. Then take a big step to the right and do a side lunge. Finish off the semicircle with a backwards lunge, then return to standing. And all that is just one rep! Aim for 10 reps and then switch legs.

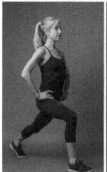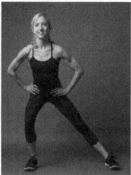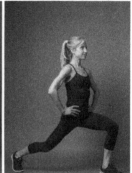

Jump Power Lunges

Stand with your feet together and lunge forward with your right foot. Jump straight up, propelling your arms. While in the air, switch legs and land in a lunge with the opposite leg forward. Repeat and continue switching legs. Try to do 10 reps. Work your way into this move gradually. It is an advanced exercise that will help you build explosive power and cardiovascular strength.

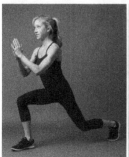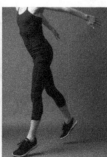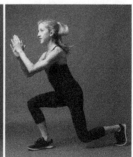

Squat

Stand with your feet hip distance apart, toes facing straight forward. Extend your arms out in front of you for balance. Sit your butt back and down, bringing your thighs parallel to the floor. Make sure your heels stay on the floor and your chest is lifted. Keep your knees behind your toes, as shown in picture. Press

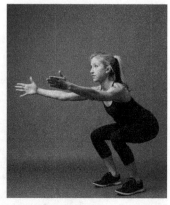

through your heels to return to a standing position.

Single Leg Squat

Stand with feet hip distance apart and raise your right leg, flexing your right ankle and pushing your hips back. Lower your body while keeping your right leg raised (a squat with one leg). Hold and then return to standing. You can use a bench to squat/sit on to work your way toward doing the single leg squat if needed. Keep your knees behind your toes and your heels firmly on the floor.

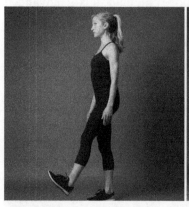
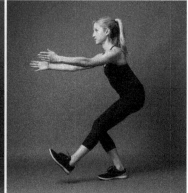

Squat Jump

This is a cardio squat! With feet hip distance apart, perform a normal squat and then jump up in the air, reaching your arms straight overhead or back behind you. Aim for 10 to 15 reps. Take a quick breather before the next set.

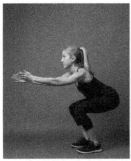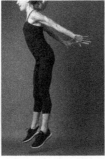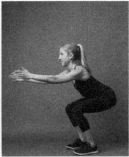

Chair Squat

Stand with feet and knees together. Sit your hips down and back as if you are sitting in a chair. Hold for 30-60 seconds or alternate lowering and lifting the hips. For more challenge, extend arms over head.

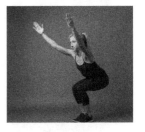

Step-Up

Find a step or bench and place your right foot on the elevated surface. Step up until your right leg is straight and then return to start. Repeat, aiming for 10-12 reps on each side. To add challenge, bring your left knee into your chest or hold weights in your hands.

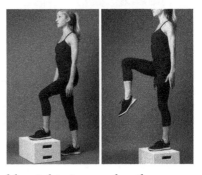

Single Leg Deadlift

Start in a standing position with feet together. Standing on your left leg, lift your right leg off the floor and bring your knee up toward your chest. Lean your upper body forward and reach your right leg out behind you. Bring your knee back up toward your chest and repeat. Perform 10-15 reps on one leg and then switch legs. Add variety by moving your arms in a running motion or bringing your arms close to the floor, deepening the lunge.

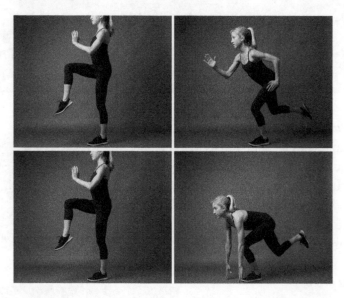

Calf Raise

From a standing position, slowly rise up on your toes, keeping your knees straight and heels off the floor. Hold briefly, then come back down. You can also try standing on something elevated (like a step) to achieve a wider range of motion.

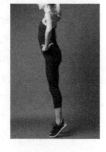

Upper Body Exercises

Push-Up

Place your hands firmly on the ground, directly under shoulders. Ground your toes into the floor to stabilize your lower half. Brace your core, engage glutes and hamstrings, and flatten your back so your entire body is neutral and straight. Lower your body. Begin to lower your body—keeping your back flat and eyes focused about three feet in front of you to keep a neutral neck—until your chest grazes the floor. Don't let your butt dip or stick out at any point during the move; your body should remain in a straight line from head to toe. Draw shoulder blades back and down, keeping elbows tucked close to your body (don't "T" your arms). Push back up keeping your core engaged; exhale as you push back to the starting position. To modify, drop knees to the floor or do a push-up standing against a wall. Repeat for 10 to 20 reps or as many as can be performed with good form.

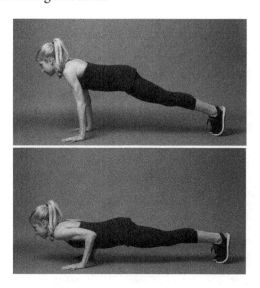

Reverse Fly

For DIY dumbbells, grab two cans or bottles of water. Bring your feet together. Hinge at your hips and bring your torso forward. Keep your knees slightly bent and engage your core. With palms facing each other and your abs engaged, extend arms out to the side, squeezing your shoulder blades. Keep your shoulders down and focus on working your upper back muscles. Repeat.

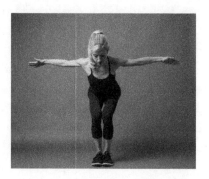

Superman

Lie facedown with arms and legs extended. With your core tight, simultaneously raise the arms and legs to form a small curve in the body. Keep your shoulders down and neck in neutral.

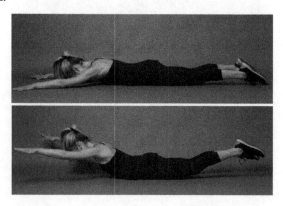

Contralateral Limb Raises, aka "Swimming"

Lie on your stomach with the arms reaching forward. Lift one arm and the opposite leg a few inches off the floor. Hold the position, then switch sides. It should feel like swimming. Use your core and keep your shoulders back and down.

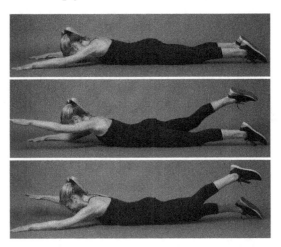

Triceps Dip

Sit on a step or bench. With knees slightly bent grab the edge of the elevated surface and straighten your arms. Bend them to a 90-degree angle, and straighten again while the heels push toward the floor. For an extra challenge, perform the exercise with straight legs or reach your right arm out while lifting your left leg.

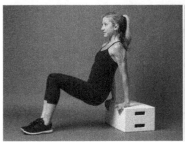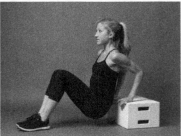

Diamond Push-Up
Follow the same guidelines as the push-up, with hands in a diamond-shaped position (situate them so that your thumbs and index fingers touch). This variation will give your triceps some extra (burning) love.

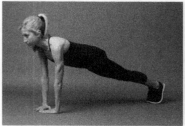 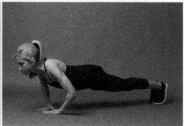

Boxer
Starting with feet hip-width apart and knees bent, keep the elbows in and punch one arm forward and the other arm back. Hug the arms back in and switch arms—like you're boxing. This one counts as cardio, strength, and core. It's also a great exercise to do to fight off fight stress if you have a few minutes to box it out at the office or at home.

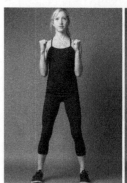 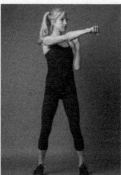 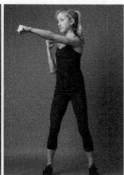

Shoulder Stabilization Series (I, Y, T, W O)

Lie down on your stomach with arms extended overhead and palms facing each other. Move your arms into an "I", a "Y", and a "T". Keep your shoulders away from your ears and keep your core engaged.

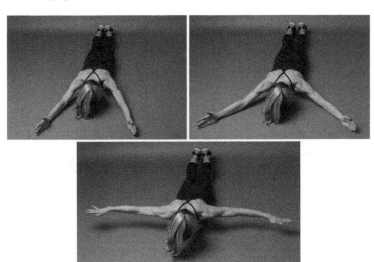

Total Body Exercises

Inchworm

Stand up tall with your legs straight. Bend at your hips and bring your fingers to touch the floor. Keep your legs straight with your knees slightly bent, and then walk your hands forward, bringing yourself to plank position. Once in a plank, start taking tiny steps so your feet meet your hands. Continue inching forward and back for 4-6 reps. This exercise is a great warm-up move before a workout or a great way to energize your whole body throughout your day.

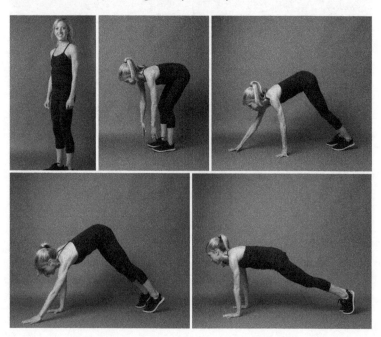

Stair Climb with Grocery Carry

Turn stairs into a cardio machine—no magic wand necessary. Grab dumbbells or household objects (bags of groceries work well) and briskly walk up and down the stairs while simulta- neously holding weight with good posture, to work your whole body. You can choose to do this exercise without equipment as well. Keep your shoulders down and back, chest open, and get your heart pumping.

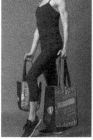
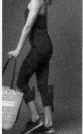

Mountain Climber

Starting in plank position, bring your left foot forward directly under your chest while straightening your right leg. Keeping your hands on the ground and core tight, switch legs. Your left leg should now be extended behind your body with your right knee forward. Continue to alternate for 30-60 seconds or 12-20 reps. Add variety with a twist, by bringing your opposite knee to your shoulder.

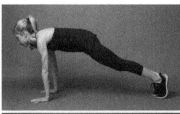
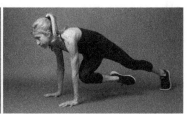
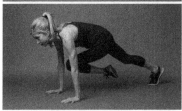

Prone Walkout

Begin by standing with your core engaged, and slowly walk your body out into a plank position. From plank, move your hands forward into a "Y," staying on your toes. Stabilize your shoulders and fire up your core as you hold. Then, gradually walk your hands back to the starting plank, maintaining your stability and balance. Only go as far as you feel comfortable and can perform in good form with stable shoulders.

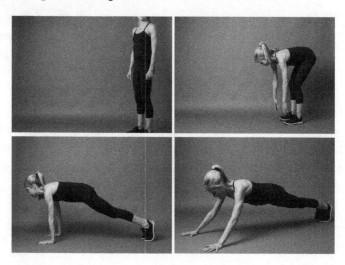

Burpees

One of the most effective full-body exercises around, and one of my favorite ways to move.

Begin in a standing position with your feet shoulder-width apart. Lower your body into a squatting position, placing your hands on the floor in front of you. Kick your feet back so that you are in push-up position. If you are new to burpees or uncomfortable kicking your feet back you can walk back into the push-up position. Lower your chest to do a push-up. Bring your chest back up. Kick your feet back to their original position. Alternately, you can walk back into the original position.

Stand up, and then jump into the air while clapping your arms overhead. Leap up as high as possible before you repeat. Do 15 reps to complete one set. If you are new to burpees, start off with 5 burpees in a row. Add challenge by using a timed interval or a variety of reps.

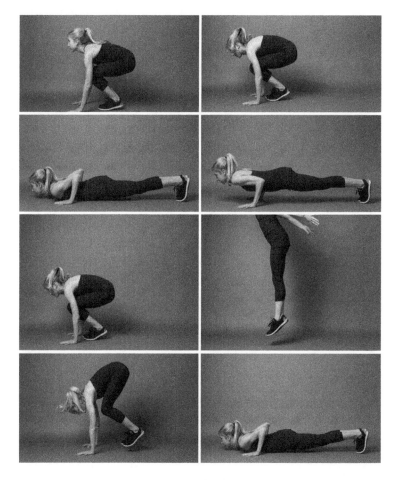

Movement exists everywhere if you look for it! Think outside the box and get active! Let exercise be your ally in living a healthy, energetic, and powerful life.

PUTTING IT ALL TOGETHER: CREATING A WEEKLY FITNESS PLAN

Learn enough about fitness, and you'll probably decide that the answer to just about every question starts with the same two words: *it depends*. Every person and situation is unique, and there is more than one way to achieve any goal. That's why this chapter provides you with basic principles and general guidelines, not unbreakable commandments.

A solid exercise program requires 30 minutes a day. That is the minimum amount of time it takes to see health benefits. You should aim to do aerobic exercise three times each week combined with at least two days of strength training and a few minutes of flexibility training. Sound like a lot? It isn't. That's only 180 minutes out of all 10,080 minutes in a week. You can totally do that.

Can this vary? Absolutely. Your program is whatever you can fit into your life consistently. Consistency is probably the most critical goal as you continue to pursue living in balance and beating burnout. That's why I advocate for short daily workouts rather than occasional long ones—the more consistent you are with healthy habits, the more successful you'll be. It is more important to make exercise a regular part of your life rather than beat yourself up over how long you spend at it.

Remember: this program is to help make you feel better. Don't allow your eating and exercise routines to increase your stress level. This will only make you feel unhappy and burdened instead of healthy. It is better to do what you feel you can do, instead of beating yourself up for not fitting another thing into an already overbooked schedule. I always say, "If it's stressing you out, you are doing it wrong." Do the best you can with what you have and build from there.

Now, let's design a fitness schedule based on your unique needs, ability level, and goals. Take 5 minutes at the start of your week to map out your workouts on your calendar. Take into account your goals, the time you have to exercise, and the workouts you enjoy most. To get the maximum health benefits, you want the following, at a minimum:

30 minutes of cardiovascular training, 3 times per week
30 minutes of strength training, 2 times per week
5–10 minutes of stretching/self-massage, daily

If you are looking for somewhere to start, plan for aerobic exercise Monday, Wednesday, and Friday and strength training for Tuesday and Thursday. That leaves the weekend for other active pursuits or to make up a workout you missed during the week. Here are examples of weekly workout schedules.

Sample Workouts

Sample Workout 1

Monday	12:00–12:30 p.m.	30-minute outdoor walk at lunch
Tuesday	6:00–6:30 p.m.	30-minute strength-training video at home after work
Wednesday	6:00–6:30 p.m.	30-minute outdoor walk after work
Thursday	6:00–6:30 p.m.	30-minute strength-training video at home after work

Friday	12:00–12:30 p.m.	30-minute outdoor walk at lunch

Sample Workout 2

Monday	6:30–7:15 a.m.	20-minute outdoor run + 5-minute abs video at home + 10 minutes of foam-rolling
Tuesday	4:30–5:30 p.m.	strength training with coach at gym
Wednesday	10-minute rest	foam roller
Thursday	6:30–7:05 p.m.	30-minute run outside after work + 5-minute stretch
Friday	6:00–7:00 p.m.	strength-training workout video at home after work
Saturday or Sunday		yoga with friends

Sample Workout 3

Monday	5:30–6:15 p.m.	45-minute spin class at gym after work
Tuesday	12:00–1:00 p.m.	60-minute lunchtime strength training
Wednesday	5:30–6:00 p.m.	30-minute jog outside after work
Thursday	5:30–6:30 p.m.	strength-training group
Friday	all day rest	

Saturday	10:00–11:00 a.m.	60-minute spin class
Sunday	7:30–8:00 p.m.	30-minute foam-rolling/ stretching

I advise planning ahead weekly for your workouts. This allows you to customize each week to your unique schedule. A habit becomes easy to perform through practice. When an action becomes easy through constant repetition, it becomes a pleasure. If it is a pleasure, it becomes second nature, and you will do it often. When a habit is part of your subconscious, it becomes a natural part of you, and then a new positive habit is born. Have you heard the saying "practice makes perfect"? It's true! I consider creating positive habits to be the most important tool I will share with you in this book. I want these positive habits to be at the center of your life. They will improve your health, activity level, energy, and attitude. I want to help teach you the habits that bring successful small changes each day and eventually lead to positive results in your life. Let me help you beat living in burnout through healthy new lifestyle habits. These positive habits are the principles that you should follow to create lasting change in your life.

If you've tried to get in shape before and it didn't work, don't worry about it. Stop dwelling on the past, and don't let the memories of old failures stop you from trying again. You've moved on, you have new tools in your hands, and the best time of your life is right around the corner.

Mapping out a weekly plan, making time to make exercise happen, and finding the right support to succeed will allow you to be consistent and see lasting results.

Your fitness is important because of the advantages to the overall physical and mental health. Fitness is about how we feel when we get up in the morning, how tired or energetic we feel after a day's work. By following the guidelines you have here, creating a fitness schedule, and sticking with it, you will know how great you feel and everyone will notice the extra pep in your step.

When you have a healthy body—one that is capable of moving well and feeling good as well as burning calories and fat efficiently—then you start to feel better about yourself. And when you feel good about yourself, your outlook on the world changes. A positive attitude and an optimistic outlook can awaken you to a wide variety of new possibilities and opportunities that self-doubt and negativity completely miss. Repeat after me: "I'm doing this for *me!*" Now get moving and be good to yourself. There is no better way to reach your goals and create positive change in your life than through exercise.

CHAPTER 3
Nutrition

Good nutrition is the fuel that will help you to beat burnout and live a life that feels good to you. Do you ever notice that some people seem to be able to fit so much more than you do into their day? They can get up, work out, go to work, take care of their kids, keep a clean house, have a hobby, and still have time to socialize? You, on the other hand, find yourself exhausted before half of the items on your to-do list are completed. If the thought of doing anything that requires more effort than sitting on the couch wears you out, I'd like you to look at the way you eat. You'd be surprised at how much more energy you can gain from a clean diet and quality nutrition.

It's all about finding balance. A lack of good food will make you weak, light-headed, and irritable. Too much food will make you sleepy or anxious, causing your body to work harder to digest it and taking away your energy and zest. When you are undernourished, you can develop chronic fatigue, depression, weight gain, and more burnout. Before this happens to you, take control and make up your mind to do something about it. Eating for energy means eating clean, eating regularly, and eating light. There is no quick-fix diet that will do what healthy eating does. And if you go "on" a diet, you'll eventually have to go "off" it, which slows your metabolism, messes with your weight, and makes you feel bad about yourself.

If you want to have a breakthrough, you need to drop the diet mind-set. Let go of the quick fix, yo-yoing, and guilt tripping, and get off the trendy eating roller-coaster. Just stop the madness. Invest in yourself: take the time to learn how to eat healthy. Adopt a way of eating that will allow you the energy and ability to enjoy living a long, full life. Healthy eating isn't as confusing, time consuming, or restrictive as you might think. The essential steps are to define your daily intake goals, eat mindfully, make smart choices, practice portion control, and water it all well with healthy hydration. When you understand and practice the basics of a healthy diet, you can stop feeling tired and start living better. Combine the suggestions offered here with your balanced body fitness program, and you'll be ready to take on any challenge with energy and enthusiasm.

Here are my guidelines for building a healthy diet and a few tools you can use to develop a way of eating that will fuel your vibrant, busy life.

LEARN WHAT YOU NEED: MINDFUL CHOICES

Define your daily intake goals (protein, carbohydrate, fat, calories), and aim to get that daily. Are you tired of feeling guilty when you eat certain foods? Are you confused about how much carbohydrate, protein, or fat you need to be your best? Do you want to make healthy diet changes but are not sure why or where to start? Taking time to learn your body's unique nutritional needs will give you the blueprint to follow to take your diet to the next healthy level. Think of your diet like a budget: when you know how much you should be spending and on what, it helps you stay on track.

Lucky for you we live in a world with many amazing tools to help guide you. There are resources that can help you define what you need, set goals, keep track of your food and physical activity, and get the nutritional details you need to be successful. You don't need to use them all—just find what works for you.

When you put the best in you can get the best out, so use these informative tools to learn how:

- USDA MyPlate. MyPlate has many features to offer. Click on different parts of the plate for a list of foods for that food group, and click on specific foods for pictures and portion sizing. This service lets you personalize a daily food plan (Daily Checklist), provides food tracking templates, and is a resource for diet analysis and planning healthy meals.
- Livestrong My Plate. This service lets you create a free profile and gives you nutritional recommendations based on your weight and activity. You can then track your diet and fitness activities to see if you are getting what you need to stay on track. Livestrong My Plate has an extensive food database for brand-specific foods and is an excellent tool for building awareness of what you are eating. There's also an active online community for sharing workouts, recipes, and motivation.
- Calorie Count. Here you can set your personal weight goal and look up nutrition facts and food labels. The phone app includes a barcode scanner for scanning in nutritional information straight from the package. It also provides nutritional analysis of food intake.

- Lose It! This tool is designed with one goal: to help you lose weight in a healthy, sustainable way. You'll find no magic pills, no crazy diets—just a simple, easy-to-use program that helps you stay within your calorie budget. The website is more comprehensive than the app and provides graphs you can use to track your weight.
- My Fitness Pal. Use the free online calorie counter and diet plan and lose weight by tracking your intake quickly and easily. Find nutrition facts for over 2,000,000 foods.

I prefer to use the Livestrong My Plate website. I can enter my personal stats (height, weight, activity level, and goals) and get guidelines on what I need each day to feel my best. Then I can enter what I'm eating and how I'm exercising each day and see if I'm on track for getting the nutrition I need to succeed. I love the pie chart that shows me the amounts of carbohydrates, proteins, and fats I am getting compared to what I need to be getting. I also can save frequently eaten foods (like my morning oatmeal) to make tracking my daily calorie intake easier. I find it really helpful in making me more mindful of how my food choices affect my nutrition, performance, and outcomes. It gives me the awareness and information I can use to continue to learn how to eat well for my needs.

Play around to uncover which tools work best for you when it comes to knowing your daily intake needs and reaching your goals. You don't need to become obsessed with these resources, but they are great for learning about calorie counts, working with portion sizes, and defining personal daily intake goals. Being equipped with the knowledge, awareness, and tools to monitor and track eating and exercise habits can be your key to success.

Take action: Define your daily nutritional needs. Aim to eat for that budget, and get the fuel you need to feel your best.

Eat Healthy (Real) Food

If I had to break down the balanced body diet into a single sentence, it would go something like this: "You're smart, and you know what real food is, so stop eating junk." You know what real food is: things that grew in the ground, on a tree, came out of the sea, moved on land, or flew through the air. Meat, fish, eggs, vegetables, fruits, and nuts are all great examples of real food.

On top of that, you know what junk food is: food that comes from a drive-thru window, vending machine, box, bag, or wrapper. If it has an ingredient list longer than a dictionary, it's probably not good for you. If it started out as real food and then went through fourteen steps to get to the point where you're about to eat it, it's probably not good for you.

Our world makes it all to easy too order pizza or reach for candy when you are busy, but if you eat junk you feel like junk. And eating poorly actually causes more stress because it takes extra effort for your body to digest junk food. If you want energy to fuel your days, use your smarts and eat real food. Not only will that help you achieve more, but it also will boost your mood and give your skin a healthy glow. If you feed your body well, it serves you well. When your body is properly nourished, you'll have sufficient energy to achieve all your goals (and then some). Nourish your body with intention, instead of indulging your appetite or feeding your emotions. Your diet should fuel you with energy and power to take on whatever life throws at you.

Take action: Bring awareness to the ingredients in the foods you are eating. How many are whole, unprocessed, and allow you to meet your daily intake goals? What processed foods can you replace with real food substitutes?

LEARN HOW MUCH YOU NEED: MINDFUL PORTIONS

Knowing how much to eat is an important key to weight loss and weight maintenance, and it's a simple skill to achieve. Eating appropriate portions enables us to eat to a point where we are comfortably full, yet not so stuffed that we regret it later. Research has shown that Americans often underestimate how many calories they consume each day by as much as 25 percent. The hard truth is that you can't outrun a bad diet. The effects of poor nutrition and over-generous portions will catch up with you at some point.

Maybe you already eat well but are unable to lose weight or gain energy due to the size of your portions. Perhaps you struggle with an all-or-nothing mentality: one chip turns into the whole bag or having a single portion is not possible with specific trigger foods. Let's work on that together! To better understand how to work well with portion sizes, you'll need to learn these three things:

- How much constitutes a portion size
- What that portion size looks like
- How to apply this knowledge in your life

The following lists include a examples of various types of food, their typical portion sizes, and everyday objects that equate to portion size. Although I include a few exceptions, most foods listed are whole foods (there is no way to include the infinite number of processed or packaged foods that are available). Since eating whole foods is always recommended over processed foods, it seems most appropriate to focus on them.

Guide to Portion Size of Whole Foods

Fresh Fruit = 1 cup = woman's fist*
- apple
- apricots
- blackberries
- blueberries
- kiwi (2)
- orange
- pear
- plums (2)
- raspberries
- strawberries
- tangerines (2)
- * Exceptions: banana, grapefruit = ½ fruit

Leafy Vegetables = 1 cup = baseball
- arugula
- baby romaine
- Boston lettuce
- mixed greens
- red lettuce
- romaine
- spinach

Fibrous Vegetables = ½ cup = ½ baseball
- artichoke hearts
- asparagus
- broccoli
- carrots
- cauliflower
- celery
- cucumber
- eggplant
- green beans
- onions
- red cabbage
- red peppers
- snap peas
- squash
- zucchini

Breads = 1 slice = CD case
- bagel (¼)
- English muffin (½)
- Whole-grain bread (1)

Meat/Protein = 3 ounces = deck of cards
- beef
- chicken breast
- pork tenderloin
- tofu
- turkey breast

Fish = 3 ounces = computer mouse
- cod
- halibut
- mahimahi

- red snapper
- salmon
- swordfish
- tuna

Grains, Legumes, Starches = ½ cup = ½ baseball
- barley (cooked)
- beans
- brown rice (cooked)
- cereal
- corn (cooked)
- edamame
- oats (cooked)
- potatoes (all varieties)
- quinoa (cooked)
- whole grain pasta (cooked)

Dairy
- hard cheese = 1.5 ounces = 4 dice or lipstick case
- yogurt = ½ cup = ½ baseball

Fats
- avocado = ½ medium = deck of cards
- oils = 1 teaspoon = 1 die
- nuts = ¼ cup = golf ball

If you don't already have measuring cups or spoons, purchase them. You may want to consider investing in a small food scale, which will allow you to weigh various foods. Compare what you are currently eating to some of the visual cues listed above. Try displaying some of the everyday items in your kitchen so you can start to learn what the right size looks like—for example, put your chicken breast next to that deck of cards.

Eventually, you'll be comfortable assessing portion sizes without measuring cups, spoons, or props and will be able to do so no matter where you are.

Knowing proper portion sizes is only half the battle in learning the art of eating the right amount. It's what you do with that knowledge that really counts. Eating out and busy schedules can make portion control more challenging. Here are my suggestions about how to use your portion control smarts in the moment.

Before eating, divide the plate.
To portion a plate properly, divide it in half. Fill one side with fruits or vegetables, leaving the rest for equal parts of protein and starch. This way, you begin to see what a properly balanced meal looks like. Spaghetti and meatballs? Steak and potatoes? They're only half a meal: incomplete without fruits and vegetables.

Pre-portion any temptations.
People tend to consume more when they have easy access to food. The bigger the package, the more food you'll pour out of it. Measure and store foods in single-serving portions. Put away all but one portion when you're ready to prepare your meal or snack, and then sit down to enjoy the right amount. I struggle with eating too many nuts, so I use this strategy to pre-portion a snack bag in advance so I don't eat 700 calories without knowing it.

Avoid mindless munching.
It's too easy to keep eating food when it's readily available. I call it the "see food diet." Many of my corporate clients struggle with this, since food is everywhere all the time at the

office—even if the foods are healthy, they gain 10 pounds from eating all the time.

You don't need to eat at all hours of the day, but if you are surrounded by food it's hard to walk away. If you can't resist food when it's around you, arrange to have it put away or leave the room. Turn off the television, computer, or any other distractions so that you can pay attention to what you are eating.

When you are dining out, ask the server to have the bread removed from the table. In the office, steer clear of your co-worker's candy jar or the community food table. Try to eliminate situations in which you'll be tempted to eat food just because it's there. If food is a constant at your office, talk to your co-workers. Tell them about your healthy living goals and see if there's a way to limit the food options to only be available at meal time. Many of them might share similar goals and would appreciate someone taking action in removing temptation.

Downsize the dishes.

If you're part of the "clean plate club" and one of the 54 percent of Americans who eat until their plates are polished, you'll want to make sure your dishware is modestly sized. On a standard 8- to 10-inch dinner plate, a portion of spaghetti looks like a meal. On a 12- to 14-inch dinner plate, it looks meager, so you're likely to dish out a bigger portion to fill the plate. Look for dishware that helps you stick to your healthy portion control goal. That way even if you eat until your plate is clean, it won't do too much damage.

Limit your choices.

The more options you have, the more options you'll want to eat. Look to limit your food choices to avoid the temptation to sample everything in sight. When at a buffet or party with a large assortment of food, view all the dining options first and then fill your plate with portions of the foods that you want most. Avoid the temptation to go back for seconds once you are comfortably full.

If you have good food in your fridge, you'll eat good food. You control 100 percent of the food that is brought into your home. Use this power to your advantage. Stock up on foods that nourish you, and if you know you can't stop at just one potato chip, then don't buy any.

Enjoy dining out with moderation and mindfulness.
Eating appropriate portion sizes when dining out is especially challenging. Restaurant serving sizes are often enough for four people. To keep portions in perspective, consider ordering two appetizers instead of an entrée. If you are dining with others, you may want to split an appetizer and entrée with another person. If you order an entrée for yourself, evaluate how much of the food on the plate equates to a portion size, then set aside the rest. You can ask for a doggie bag and save the portion for another meal during the week. If you choose to have dessert, share it! You can have a few bites, satisfy your sweet tooth, and still honor your goals.

LEARN WHEN YOU ARE HUNGRY: MINDFUL EATING

"Am I hungry?" Before eating, learn to check in with yourself and separate physical hunger from emotional hunger. Are you really hungry? Or are you just stressed, tired, anxious, or over-whelmed? Listening to your body's physical cues will help you learn how to eat when you are hungry, stop when you are full, and respect your body's needs.

If you find that you are not hungry and are eating for emotional reasons, start by raising your awareness of when you are vulnerable to emotional eating. Write down where and when you eat or drink due to stress. The office? Late at night? When you are alone? Do you notice any patterns? Every time before you eat, ask yourself how physically hungry you are on a scale of 1 to 10. If you are a 6 to a 10, it's likely that you are physically hungry. But if you are a 3, it might signify that you are eating in response to your emotions and may be better off with two minutes of deep breathing or something else that helps you cope with your emotions. (See part III, Balanced Mind, for ideas). Above all, the keys are mindfulness and empowering yourself to choose healthier habits instead of trying to "eat" your feelings. Be aware of falling into the trap of soothing and comforting yourself with food. Know that you are in control. You have a choice, always. If you want to put an end to emotional eating, you can do it by building awareness and working to create healthier, stress-relieving habits.

Spend your mealtime as sacred time for yourself. Eating is an act of nourishing your body, separating yourself from work, and allowing yourself time to replenish and regroup. Practice having meals away from your desk, TV, smartphone, or other distractions. Enjoy healthy food with people you love, a little reading, people watching, or chatting with a friend. Multitasking for work while eating is never productive. Break the habit, and give yourself a meal break that's good for your mind and body.

Plan Your Meals

Eating well starts with planning ahead and having an eating blueprint. To successfully eat well, you have to think ahead and make time to prepare or get healthy meals. This doesn't need to be a crazy or intense process; it's just about having an idea of what you are going to eat and when. Even if your idea of pre-planning is getting healthy food to go from the Whole Foods Market salad bar, it's better than leaving it to chance and getting stuck without healthy options when mealtime comes. When you are hungry, it's much harder to make healthy choices. You don't need much time—just a commitment to think ahead. Having healthy foods stocked and a plan of what you want to eat will make it easy to honor your diet goals. Many people get overwhelmed at the thought of meal planning, or they make it overly complicated. Don't overthink it! Just write out when, where, and what you plan to eat, and schedule a time to shop (or use a service) so that you have what you need. Here are some amazing resources you can use to get inspired, plan your meals, and prepare for success.

Resources for Healthy Meal Planning, Recipes, and Menus

Eatingwell.com
Free diet and meal plans, weekly menus, healthy recipes, and grocery shopping lists for every dietary preference and calorie budget. This content-rich website is full of information and inspiration to fuel your healthy lifestyle. I love the weekly menus and use the clean recipes often.

Cookinglight.com
Find quick and healthy recipes, nutrition tips, entertaining menus, and fitness guides to help you cook and live lightly.

Myrecipes.com/healthy-diet
Thousands of healthy recipes plus nutrition news, diet recipes, and smart cooking strategies for a healthy diet. This website is

fantastic because it combines great, healthy, calorie-conscious recipes with coverage of new health studies and tips for reaching your weight-loss goals. It also includes vegetarian meals, diabetic recipes, and meals for other specialty diets. You'll find lots of information and encouragement for healthy eating without compromising flavor.

The following healthy-meal delivery services can support your healthy eating goals. To check if these services are available near you, do a Web search for "healthy meal delivery" or "healthy grocery delivery." You might find similar services in your area that are equal to or better than these options.

Instacart.com
If you are too busy to grocery shop, use a service to do it for you. Instacart is a website with a smartphone app that lets you order your groceries and have them delivered to your doorstep.

Zesty.com
The website and smartphone app for this meal delivery service make it easy for you and your company to eat healthy, delicious food. Curated by in-house dietitians, Zesty delivers fresh dishes from your favorite local restaurants.

Munchery.com
Use this meal delivery service online or your smartphone app. Munchery answers "What's for dinner?" with nourishing, affordable, chef-cooked meals delivered right to your door. Local chefs make meals—including healthy, tempting kids' meals—with fresh, seasonal ingredients that are sourced from local, organic sources as much as possible. Dishes are fully cooked, chilled for maximum freshness, and served in oven- and microwave-safe containers for easy heating in fewer

than 10 minutes. Both on-demand and scheduled delivery are available.

Cooksmarts.com

Cook Smarts isn't so much a website and app as it is an entire meal planning service. In addition to helping you plan your weekly meals, the service aims to help its users learn to cook, explore new recipes, get familiar with and comfortable in the kitchen, and eat more healthy, homemade food. The site's blog and newsletter are free, but to make use of their meal planning tools, you'll have to sign up for an account. You can get three sample plans for free, but the service will cost you $6 to $8 per month. The meal plans themselves are incredibly robust, though; you tell the service how you want to eat—vegetarian, high protein, low carb, paleo, or a simple balanced diet—and you'll get four new and interesting recipes every week, along with ingredients, a downloadable and printable grocery list, and step-by-step instructions and cooking videos to help you make everything.

Of course these are just a few of the options available to you. There are many, many websites that provide healthy alternatives to heavier dishes and tips to make a healthy diet not just a temporary fix but an ongoing lifestyle.

Breakfast: How You Start Your Day Is How You Live It

Are you too busy for breakfast? Not hungry for a meal in the morning? An only-coffee-till-noon kind of worker? Well, you are doing your body a huge disservice by skipping out. Many miss breakfast to try to save time or even believe that eliminating breakfast will help them lose weight. Wrong! Skipping a morning meal will actually slow you down and make maintaining a healthy weight more difficult. Nobody's body or brain likes going without fuel till lunchtime; failing to eat breakfast will force your system into starvation mode and cause your metabolism to shut down. Even if you don't feel hungry, a little bit of nutrition in the morning goes a long way. Making time for breakfast and creating a morning meal habit could quite possibly be the routine that helps you maintain a healthy weight, feel great, and power up to kick butt. Here are a few reasons a healthy breakfast is a must.

Breakfast kick-starts the metabolism.
Eating breakfast speeds up your metabolism, thereby helping you to burn more calories rather than store them as fat.

Breakfast boosts nutrient intake.
Breakfast eaters have a higher fiber intake and significantly higher intake of vitamins and minerals, especially calcium, iron, and magnesium—that is, of course, if you choose to eat a nutritious breakfast rather than a coffee shop muffin.

Breakfast helps prevent binge eating.
Have you ever gone too long without eating and then over-eaten at the next opportunity? Eating a balanced breakfast will help regulate your hunger, keep blood sugar levels stable, and prevent you from bingeing on sugar, processed carbs, or other unhealthy foods. It also will help you end the late-night eating habit that keeps so many from achieving their weight goals.

Breakfast improves memory and concentration.
People who eat a healthy breakfast concentrate better, are more efficient, and have an improved mood, in comparison to

those who skip breakfast. Makes sense: when your brain gets fuel, it uses it for power.

Breakfast helps you maintain your weight.
People who eat breakfast are more likely to maintain a healthy weight.

All these reasons should help you see why breakfast is essential in boosting metabolism, preventing bingeing, and improving your body's ability to perform. It doesn't take a lot to create a breakfast habit; in fact, you can whip up a fabulous morning meal in less than 5 minutes. There are many fast and easy breakfast options that don't require a lot of prep work or effort. Here are a few nutritious ideas to get you started on brainstorming what might work for you.

Fast and Fabulous Healthy Breakfast Ideas to Power You Up for Your Busy, Successful Life

Overnight Oatmeal

I make this the night before, and it's ready to go in the morning. I'm addicted and love all my flavorful toppings. Here is my go-to oatmeal recipe.

Caroline's Growing Oatmeal Bowl
Serving: 1 happy breakfast bowl

- ½ cup gluten-free oats
- ¼ teaspoon salt
- 1½ cups water or milk of choice

- 1 tablespoon chia seeds
- Preferred sweetener (I add a packet or two of stevia)
- Add-ins of choice

1. Place your oats and salt in a large pot with the liquid of choice. (You can use all water, but it's much creamier with milk. I often use a combination of water and almond milk.)
2. Bring water to a boil and simmer mixture for 1½ minutes.
3. Turn off heat and add chia seeds.
4. Stir, seal the lid of the pot, and then allow to sit and soak overnight.

When you jump out of bed in the morning, the oatmeal will be thick and ready for your favorite add-ins. It's really amazing how much it increases in volume overnight. Sometimes I even add another ½ cup liquid and heat it up a bit in the morning for a softer, warmer bowl of oats.

If you don't want to wait overnight for the oatmeal, try the same recipe, cooking for 12–15 minutes, stirring often. This should make a very thick and creamy bowl of oatmeal.

Now for the fun part: toppings. Here are a few of my favorites:

- Fresh fruit
- Dried fruit: raisins, figs, apricots
- Nuts: pecans, almonds, walnuts
- Seeds: sunflower, pumpkin
- Dried coconut
- Jam
- Cinnamon
- Almond or vanilla extract
- Freeze-dried fruit (mango is surprisingly addictive)
- Vanilla protein powder

After all is said and done, eat, enjoy, and smile a ton!

Other Breakfast Favorites

- Sliced banana mixed with 2 tablespoons of almond butter and a sprinkling of toasted shredded coconut
- Natural yogurt with a sliced apple, berries, and a teaspoon of ground flaxseeds
- Green protein smoothie
  Try this simple apple protein smoothie: Combine one scoop protein powder with one apple, a handful of spinach, water, or almond milk, and your preferred sweetener to taste. Blend in a blender and enjoy!
- Blackberries mixed with ricotta, ½ teaspoon honey, and grated lemon zest
- Swiss muesli
  Combine 2 cups rolled oats and 1 cup milk (your choice). Cover and refrigerate overnight. In the morning, add 2 grated apples, ¼ cup chopped hazelnuts, 8 ounces plain yogurt, and a drizzle of honey. Mix well. Serves 4.
- Egg whites + ½ avocado + berries (Takes 15 minutes, and it's amazing!)
- Toast + avocado + tomatoes, another quick, out-the-door meal
- Sliced tomatoes topped with cheese and grilled, served with a hard-boiled egg
- An egg fried in coconut oil and served with sautéed mushrooms, tomatoes, and spinach
- Large lettuce leaf filled with grilled bacon, a little cottage cheese, tomatoes and spinach and rolled up
- Fruit smoothie

Blend a handful of berries, half a frozen banana, a large handful of spinach, and a cup of milk with 1 teaspoon ground flaxseeds

- Dried fruit and mixed nuts
  If you aren't hungry in the morning or are on the go, this may be a good option for you. Put one serving in a plastic bag and eat on the way to work with a thermos of milk, green juice, etc.
- Breakfast burrito with scrambled eggs, chopped tomatoes (or salsa), and a little grated cheese, wrapped in a big lettuce leaf
- Cottage cheese mixed with sliced fresh pineapple
- Kippers or smoked salmon with cooked tomatoes, mushrooms, and onions
- Fresh figs halved and wrapped in prosciutto slices
- Scrambled tofu in a little olive oil, with onions, peppers, and a dash of light soy sauce; with a small bowl of mixed berries
- Lean ham or turkey rolled up in a lettuce leaf with grated cheese and a dollop of salsa
- Sliced melon tossed in a bowl with the pulp of one passionfruit and topped with plain yogurt and a handful of chopped nuts
- Protein "blobs"
  In a bowl or food processor, combine 1 cup unsweetened, unsalted peanut butter, 4 scoops whey protein powder, 1 teaspoon vanilla extract. Form the mixture into balls and roll them in crushed nuts or coconut (optional). Makes about 14.
- Vanilla chia pudding
  In a jar with a tight-fitting lid, combine a 13.5-ounce can of coconut milk, 4 tablespoons honey, 1 teaspoon vanilla extract, and ¼ teaspoon cinnamon. Shake vigorously. Then,

add ¼ cup chia seeds and shake again. Place in the fridge and wait roughly 30 minutes for the mixture to set. Make the night before for a quick breakfast in the morning.

If you think you feel good without breakfast, imagine how great you'll feel with it. Carve out 5 minutes in the evening to prep a nutritious breakfast for yourself. Grab and go and you are out the door with more energy than a superhero.

All Natural Snacks for Energy and Health

Your days are nonstop, and sometimes you need a little extra oomph between meals. That's when having a healthy snack on hand can be powerful. Healthy snacks can absolutely be a part of your balanced body diet. You just need to do it right, and no, I'm sorry, Cheetos don't count. Remember: junk snacks will make you feel like junk! You deserve to feel good, so let's make snack choices that support that. Some of the healthiest options are plant based, gluten free, dairy free, and sugar free. In other words, they're all-natural bites that don't contain any of the anti-nutrients that rob your body of energy and decrease your ability to function at your best. Healthy snacking can help you maintain stable blood sugar levels, give you energy to fuel your day, and prevent you from reaching for sugar when you want an energy boost. Here are some of the best things to eat to keep your mind and body fueled with all day energy.

Green juice
This is the ultimate energy booster. Green vegetable juice is loaded with antioxidants, phytonutrients, chlorophyll, magnesium, and potassium. Your cells instantly gobble up these nutrients, making you feel energized and alert. Make sure the

green juice is from vegetables and is not a fruit juice disguised as a green juice. Aim to keep the carbohydrate content below 20 grams; above this amount, the juice is too sugary and may cause blood sugar fluctuations and energy drops.

Nuts or natural trail mix

Nuts are an easy way to get a delicious dose of protein in a convenient, shelf-stable package. Try a mixed bunch for variety and a combo with dried fruit for some added sweetness. Nuts are calorically dense and full of nutrients, so put some serving-size portions in plastic baggies so you don't accidentally overdo it. Looking for the best bang for your protein buck? Almonds and pistachios are higher in protein than their nutty peers.

It doesn't get much easier than trail mix. Toss together your favorite nuts, dried fruits, and other tasty items. Just watch the portion size to avoid overdoing it on snack calories.

Whole fruit

Known as nature's original prepackaged snack, you can't beat fruit for its portability, nutrients, and wonderful sweet taste. The following fruits are favorites for school and work snacks: bananas, apples, peaches, nectarines, plums, grapes, blueberries, and raspberries.

Fresh fruit salad

This will keep for a few hours in your lunch bag, but if you have refrigeration available, that's better. Put any of the following in some portable containers: diced mango, pineapple chunks, melon balls (watermelon, honeydew, or cantaloupe), berries, grapes, and kiwi.

Dried or dehydrated fruit

When you need some energy foods with a longer shelf life, dried fruit is very handy. For straight-up snacking, these are my top picks: blueberries, raisins, cranberries, apricots, and mulberries. I've also recently gotten into goji berries for the incredible energy they produce and their health benefits.

All-natural bars

When you're on the run, faced with limited choices, traveling, or simply craving more snack variety, a quality bar can help you curb hunger and maintain energy. Look for a bar with whole food ingredients, around 10 grams of protein, and less than 15 grams of sugar. Some of my favorites include Larabars, Vega Protein bars, Aloha protein bars, Kind bars, Health Warrior bars, and Go Macro bars.

Protein powder

Keep a stash of packets or baggies of protein powder to mix into water or juice when you are on the go. Some dairy-free brands come in a variety of flavors. When you are in a hurry you can mix up the protein powder in a bottle with water or milk of your choice. If you have more time, blend up the protein powder with an apple or some other produce to make it more filling and delicious.

Apple butter on a rice cake

Since apple butter doesn't actually contain butter, it is naturally gluten and casein free. I put it on organic rice cakes that are also gluten free.

Peanut butter and pretzels

You can make this an allergen-free snack with gluten- or wheat-free pretzels and single-serving packs of nut butter.

Nut or seed butter with sliced apples
To up the flavor, stir a little cinnamon and/or vanilla into the nut butter. If you're bored with peanut butter and almond butter, then sample cashew butter or seed butter.

Hummus with cut veggies
Hummus is one snack food I can never get enough of. I pair it with baby carrots, celery, broccoli, cauliflower, and sliced red bell peppers.

Hummus with olives and crackers or pita chips

Smashed avocado with baby carrots
To keep the avocado from browning, mix in some lemon or lime juice. You can even season to taste with salt and spices for a quick guacamole to go.

Canned wild salmon salad with crackers or lettuce wraps
Tuna works well too, but salmon gives you the extra omega-3s.

Hard-boiled eggs
Enjoy this perfect protein on the go. Sprinkle with a little salt, pepper, and paprika for a tasty twist.

Grilled chicken breast
At only 110 calories, 1.5 grams of fat, and 25 grams of protein, this is a low-calorie, protein-packed snack.

Jerky
Seek out organic and all-natural options.

Dates stuffed with almonds
Yum!

Apple chips
Made from slices of real, fresh apples and 90–100 calories per serving, this delicious snack should be free of preservatives, trans fats, cholesterol, and refined sugar. It's a great source of dietary fiber and is gluten free, vegan, and kosher.

Edamame
One cup offers a whopping 17 grams of protein.

That's a lot of ideas to keep you snacking smart and feeling good. Plan ahead and prep some healthy options to pack with you and place in your office fridge, gym bag, or shelves at home. Use Amazon Prime, Google Shopping Express, or Instacart to help you stay stocked when your schedule is too busy for a grocery store trip. A little planning goes a long way and can keep you healthy, happy, and energized from quality nutrition.

THE 80/20 RULE

While healthy eating is important, there are times when we all want to indulge and need a little wiggle room to do so. Life is meant to be enjoyed, and if having a piece of cake at your friend's birthday party is going to bring you pleasure, then by all means you should have a piece of cake. That's why I subscribe to the 80/20 rule. This rule reminds you that if you want to maintain a healthy body and weight, you'll need to make wise food choices more often than not, but you can make occasional allowances for certain foods or larger portion sizes without falling off track. Depriving yourself to an extreme isn't sustainable long term, and neither is indulging 24/7. When you don't let yourself enjoy what you love, you end up craving them more. This is where practicing moderation comes in. Moderation allows you to enjoy some of the sweeter and more savory foods without overdoing them or sabotaging your efforts to maintain healthy habits. By indulging wisely and treating yourself once in a while, it's actually easier to stay on track and maintain a healthy life.

You don't have to be perfect or make healthy choices 100 percent of the time to be fit, strong, happy, and well. Here are my guidelines for making the 80/20 rule work in your life.

Be choosy.

Part of indulging wisely is figuring out what is really worth the indulgence and what splurging means to you. For instance, if you have a sweet tooth but can take or leave French fries or potato chips, save your indulgences for dessert. When you're confronted with unhealthy foods you don't really crave or love, either skip those or substitute healthier foods so you have room later for the indulgence you really want. Let's say you dine at a restaurant, and chips or fries come with your sandwich; ask to substitute a salad, fruit, or vegetable for the chips or fries if dessert is a more appealing treat. Even some fast-casual restaurants allow you to do this. Swapping out unhealthy foods for healthier choices not only gives you more room to enjoy the things that are really worth the indulgence, but it also helps you to eat more nutritious foods along the way. Don't waste your calories on things you don't love. Use your 20 percent on what you really want.

Plan ahead for your 20 percent indulgences.

Every week, go over your schedule and pick the one day or specific moments when you want to allow yourself to enjoy the things you normally avoid. If you know you have a big event on Saturday night, that might be the perfect occasion to indulge.

If you know you have a birthday dinner with a friend on Wednesday, you might want to enjoy treats then. Regardless of the occasion or the timing, planning indulgences ahead of time gives you something to look forward to throughout the week so it's easier to remain healthy the rest of the time.

Plan the other 80 percent.
Plan your week's meals and snacks to make it easier to remain healthy 80 percent of the time. Make sure you shop for all the required ingredients and prepare to be successful in your planned meals. Think ahead, plan to succeed, and you'll build a healthy habit of 80 percent nutritious meals.

Savor your splurges.
When it's time to indulge, enjoy it. Don't let guilt get in the way or beat yourself up for having a treat. Practice awareness when eating so you maintain a healthy level of satisfaction and don't feel physically ill or overstuffed. Take the time to enjoy your treat away from TV, work, or other distractions. Slow down, be mindful, and savor every second.

Take the frequent indulgences Rx.
There will always be times when opportunities to indulge are more frequent than normal: holiday seasons, vacations, and birthdays are good examples. When this happens, the best thing you can do, as always, is plan for it. Otherwise, one celebration can easily blend into another, and before you know it you've spent a full week or two indulging over and over. Here are some ways you can offset these occasions so they don't overtake your attempts to maintain a healthy lifestyle.

Exercise

During those weeks you know you'll be indulging more than 20 percent of the time, spend some extra time moving. Even an additional 20 to 30 minutes during your workout can make a huge difference. Also choose to incorporate more movement into your day to day, taking the stairs and walking as much as possible.

Nutrition

For those times when indulging is more frequent, eat especially light and healthy when you aren't celebrating. Choose to eat nourishing whole foods and raw fibrous fruits and vegetables. Also make sure you stay hydrated. Before you indulge, drink two glasses of water to fill yourself up so you indulge a little bit less than you would otherwise.

Support

Communicate your health goals to others and recruit support to help keep you on track. For example, ask your family or friends to exercise with you or prepare healthy menu for group meals. Communicate your goals and desire to be healthy. The more open and honest you are with those who can help you, the more successful you'll be. Accountability is a highly motivating success strategy.

Reset

There will be times when your healthy habits start to wane. Accept that this is a natural part of life. Remember that every day is a new day and a new beginning. If you find yourself spiraling into unhealthier habits on a regular basis, hit the restart button. Recruit support from friends, family, or your fitness coach. Choose to regain control, and let the small setback teach you how to move forward to be your best.

The 80/20 rule is all about knowing that we need to give ourselves some wiggle room to maintain healthy eating over our lifetime. It is easy to become unmotivated if you feel like you've screwed up by not eating perfectly. All too often this is used as an excuse to continue to eat poorly. It's impossible to eat perfectly all the time. Instead, choose to drop the all-or-nothing mind-set and adopt a moderate 80/20 approach so you can make the indulgences you love a part of your life.

Don't feel guilty about a bad meal or an unhealthy weekend. Pick yourself up right where you left off as soon as you can, and continue living your life. Make small, permanent changes that you can live with until they become habit, and then pick another small change to tackle. It's all about progress, not perfection. Work on your health, your choices, and your attitude toward yourself. Consider where you want to go, recruit support, and set small realistic goals. Any small steps forward *will* add up to progress and fulfilling your vision of a healthy, balanced life.

DRINK WATER

Roughly 60 percent of the body is water. Drinking enough H_2O maintains the body's fluid balance, which helps transport nutrients in the body, regulate body temperature, digest food, and more. Most of the time, we are in a constant state of dehydration and our thirst centers are so dulled that we don't even know it. Dehydration messes with energy levels, and often the brain confuses thirst as hunger, causing you to want to eat when you really just need water. The amount of water people need per day is up for debate, but studies suggest adults need 9 to 16 cups of H_2O. However this number varies depending on activity level, age, and how much water is consumed in coffee, tea, or water-rich veggies and fruit.

Here's how to keep yourself hydrated: Begin each day by drinking a glass of water as soon as you wake up, and then 30 minutes before eating any big meal. Drinking more water is a habit you can cultivate, and it's not hard to do it. Get in the habit of keeping a water bottle on hand at all times. When it comes to beverages, water is number one, and you can also spice it up. Make it *easy* to drink well. Here are some simple lifestyle hacks for better beverage choices:

- Choose water or low-calorie beverages instead of sugar-sweetened beverages.
- For a quick, easy, and inexpensive thirst quencher, carry a water bottle and refill it throughout the day.
- Don't stock the fridge with sugar-sweetened beverages. Instead, keep a jug or bottles of cold water in the fridge.
- Serve water with meals.
- Make water more exciting by adding slices of lemon, lime, cucumber, or watermelon
- Drink sparkling water.
- Add a splash of 100 percent juice to plain sparkling water for a refreshing, low-calorie drink.
- When you do opt for a sugar-sweetened beverage, go for the small size. Some companies are now selling 8-ounce cans and bottles of soda, each of which contains about 100 calories.
- Read the ingredients on "low-calorie" or diet beverages and try to stay away from artificial ingredients and fake sweeteners.

- Be a role model for your friends and family by choosing healthy, low-calories beverages.

Take action: Bring awareness to your hydrating habits. How much water are you currently drinking per day? Is it enough to fuel your busy life? If not, it's time to create a healthy hydrating habit. Find ways to make drinking water easy for you. Get a refillable water bottle, set a phone alarm, add fruit to your water, pour a glass at every meal. Notice how different you feel with more water! Now stick with it. Your body loves you.

BODY BURNOUT AND BOOZE

Wednesday night client drinks. Thursday night charity event. Friday night birthday party. Saturday brunch. Saturday evening dinner date. Sunday brunch. Sunday night wine-and-dine with girlfriends. You have a social life, but you hate what it's doing to your health. Body and mind burnout is next on the calendar if you don't do something about it.

Too many late nights out, networking events, and alcoholic drinks can have harsh effects on your body (not to mention your mental health). While drinking alcohol and going out can fit into your balanced body lifestyle, there's one reality we just can't change: alcoholic drinks are just another source of extra, empty calories, and staying up late does not help you get your beauty sleep. Here are a few of the ways alcohol can get in the way of your health and fitness goals.

Slower recovery from workouts and long workdays
Hard workouts or challenging workdays drain the glycogen stores (carbs stored in the liver and muscles) and leave your

muscle tissue in need of repair. Pouring alcohol into your system stalls the recovery process. High levels of alcohol displace the carbs, leaving you without quality nutrition to help you recover from hard workouts or workdays.

Packed-on fat

Alcohol is an empty source of calories. When booze is on board, besides having to deal with the surplus of calories, your body prioritizes metabolizing the alcohol over burning fat and carbs. Alcohol also breaks down amino acids and stores them as fat. For some reason this process tends to be most pronounced in the thighs, stomach, and glutes. Excessive alcohol consumption really packs on poundage to those areas, hence the reason we have the term *beer belly*. Alcohol also increases levels of cortisol (a stress hormone), which further encourages fat storage, particularly in your midsection.

Disrupted sleep

Drinking and late nights also affect your muscle recovery and performance by sapping your sleep. In a study of 93 men and women, researchers found that alcohol decreased sleep duration and increased wakefulness (particularly in the second half of the night), especially in women, whose sleep time was decreased by more than 30 minutes over the night.

Depleted water and nutrients

Alcohol irritates the stomach lining, which can reduce your capacity to absorb nutrients (the reason you have an upset stomach after a few too many drinks). And alcohol makes you pee. For every gram of ethanol you suck down, you pump out 10 milliliters of urine (that's about 9.5 ounces for two beers). As little as 2 percent dehydration hurts your performance (and gives you a major headache). And no, you can't rehydrate with a dehydrating drink (e.g., beer); water is the only thing that can help you hydrate yourself back to health.

These are just a few of the many ways drinking or staying out can affect your health goals. You don't have to give up drinking or going out to live a balanced life, you just have to learn to do it smarter. Moderation is the key here. There are ways you can maintain your shape and health, even if you drink alcohol or go out. If alcohol is a part of your life, here are my suggestions for enjoying it in moderation and still honoring your goals the next morning.

Socialize SMART: Booze and Beating Burnout

Pick a few days a week when you will avoid alcohol, and stick to your plan.
Many people find it easiest to just say no drinking Monday through Thursday. Think about your life and your routine, and come up with at least three days of the week when you won't drink.

Learn to drink in moderation.
The truth is it's not possible to drink every day, or binge drink on weekends, and still be healthy. That type of drinking makes you less likely to exercise, less likely to eat healthy, and more likely to cause harm to your body (higher risk of some cancers, liver disease, metabolic problems, accidents, etc.). Plus, most of us don't need the extra calories. Think of alcohol as junk food—it's fine to indulge, just not in excess.

When you do drink, plan ahead to account for the calories.
This could mean eating extra healthy, avoiding sweets or processed foods, or scheduling in a hard workout on the day you're
going to drink. Think of each drink as about 150 non-nutri-
tious calories that you'll have to cut out elsewhere. By the way,
one drink = 5 ounces of wine (but a typical restaurant pour is 6
to 7 ounces), 12 ounces of beer (but a typical draught beer is a
pint, or 16 ounces), or 1.5 ounces of liquor.

*Choose wine, light beer, or simple cocktails made with
low-calorie mixers.*
Just as you might order your salad with dressing on the side,
don't be shy about asking for your cocktail your way. Mix cocktails with water, club soda, or low-calorie juices for easy calorie savings. Fruit and vegetable juices can be good choices
because they are lower in calories than some other mixers and
also contain disease-preventing antioxidants. Still, be careful
of fruit juices because even though they are more nutritious,
the calories can add up quickly. Some mixers that won't pack
on the pounds include these:

- Diet soda, soda water, or diet tonic: 0 calories
- Orange juice (6 oz.): 84 calories
- Cranberry juice cocktail (8 oz.): 136 calories
- Light orange juice (8 oz.): 50 calories
- Light cranberry juice (8 oz.): 40 calories
- Light lemonade (8 oz.): 5 calories
- Coffee, tea: 0 calories
- Lemon or lime juice (½ oz.): 10 calories
- Original Margarita Mix Sweet-n-Sour Mix

Skip the mixer.

Try ordering your favorite spirit or one of the new flavored liquors on the rocks. Infused vodkas are popular—they are not sweetened; they are infused with flavors (like jalapeño or peach), and don't add any extra calories.

Before you go out, decide on a set number of drinks that you will use as a limit.

If not, you'll make that same mistake over and over of having a few too many. Tell yourself, "Okay, I'll have two or three drinks throughout the whole night, and I'm good!"

Always eat a meal before you enjoy your favorite cocktails.

It's important to eat balanced, regular meals to keep your blood sugar stable and your metabolism running full speed. Eating regular meals will make you less likely to eat bar food when you are out late at night and will help you avoid a hangover from drinking.

Watch what you eat while you drink.

It's easy to let the munchies get control of you during or after you drink. And can you recall a time when you started drinking and all of a sudden you craved a salad? Me either. Snacks consumed while drinking tend to be high-calorie ones, as do the meals people eat when they're hung over. Drinking also lowers your inhibitions, so you're much more likely to overdo it on nachos and wings when you've had a few.

Alternate water with cocktails.

Drink water between cocktails to stay hydrated and avoid a hangover in the morning. Keep a 1:1 ratio of water and drinks.

Choose spritzers and lighter drink choices.
Spritzers are made with soda water and cut wine calories in half. My favorite light cocktail is a tequila soda with a splash of lime.

Don't think that because it's labeled "low-carb" or "light" that you can drink more of it.
As is true with food, if you pick the "diet" versions of drinks, it can play tricks with your mind and cause you to think you can have more of it. Wrong! Just cause it's "light" doesn't mean you can have twice the amount.

Quality vs. quantity.
Sometimes it's better just to order the real thing. Order a glass of something top shelf that you'll enjoy (red wine if you love it). You'll make it last longer and actually savor it.

Be like the French, Italians, and Greeks: sit back, have a little something, and enjoy.
In many cultures, people enjoy a daily (small) drink and are able to maintain good health and a reasonable weight.

Always have a designated driver or another form of transportation.
You do not want to risk hurting a stranger, a friend, or yourself.

Have a friend to go out with.
Dance together, keep each other in check, and make sure you are having the best time ever. You can keep each other accountable so that you don't blow all your hard work by drinking your body weight in cocktails.

Never lose track of your drink by putting it down at a party, bar, or other gathering.

You can drink plain water.
If you are not in the mood or have an early morning, order soda water with lime and enjoy yourself with friends.

Work out the next day.
It's helpful to maintain a regular workout routine, no matter how late you were out socializing. Exercise is the best energy booster and headache helper. A workout will help fight fatigue and heal the foggy morning brain from a late night out.

Look at your schedule and plan ahead.
Balance nights out within your week to avoid being out late or drinking every night. If you know you have an event on Thursday and a birthday party on Saturday, schedule down-time on Wednesday and Friday to chill, relax, and do some exercise.

Keep it classy.
Be a breath of fresh air to others. A sloppy, drunk mess is not fun, attractive, or enjoyable to be around.

Develop means of relaxation that don't include drinking.
Don't just drink to drink. Many adults get in the habit of daily drinking to relax and leave work behind. Many people also develop the habit of ordering multiple cocktails when they go out (pre-party, party, after-party—it all adds up). If you regularly drink to relax or socialize, you'll pack on the pounds. (And making a habit of it is not a good idea when it comes to alcohol.) Build awareness into your habits when it comes to alcohol. If you need alcohol to relax, think about other activities that

are relaxing and enjoyable to you—working out, taking a walk outside, listening to music, reading, and so on—and schedule those into your life as a means of unwinding instead of opening a bottle of wine every night. If you need alcohol to feel more comfortable when you are socializing, strengthen your socializing skills by *not* using alcohol to make you more comfortable. Breaking any habit is hard, especially when it comes to booze. But like anything, the more you practice, the easier it gets. And I'd rather practice enjoying the quality of my life than drinking my way through it, wouldn't you?

All that being said, when you belly up to the bar, what are the best and worst cocktail choices?

The Worst Cocktail Choices

Margarita
This one drink can have up to 750 calories and 56 grams of carbs. Substitute a tequila on the rocks with a splash of lime.

Long Island Iced Tea
A Long Island Iced Tea has about 750 calories and 44 grams of carbs. Try rum mixed with diet cola and topped with a slice of lime; it will save you more than 600 calories.

Piña Colada
The Piña Colada comes in at a whopping 650 calories and 90 grams of carbs. Substitute with vanilla-flavored vodka and diet cola or lemon–lime and you'll save more than 500 calories.

Cosmopolitan

The Cosmo may have only 150 calories and 10 grams of carbs, but this sweet drink is too easy to enjoy quickly. It's too hard not to order more, turning the cosmo into a costly cocktail. Try vodka with a splash of cranberry juice instead.

The Best Cocktail Choices

Gin and Tonic, Vodka and Tonic, or Rum and Diet Coke

All of these have only 65 calories per 8 ounces. When you drink a 1-ounce pour of most liquors and top them off with a noncalorie mixer, you have a drink that's pretty low in calories, no matter what the combination. Whether you choose gin, vodka, whiskey, or rum, top it off with a mixer that adds nothing: club soda, diet cola, or diet tonic water. Make your drink special with infused alcohol flavors, small splashes of juice, or sugar-free syrups.

Mimosa

Half champagne and half orange juice, the Mimosa is at its best when made with the freshest-squeezed juice imaginable for only 75 calories per 4 ounces.

Kahlua and Coffee

Surprisingly, at 91 calories per 6 ounces this classic cocktail can fulfill your alcohol needs and your caffeine needs with fewer calories than many other drinks. Kahlua is the most famous brand of coffee-flavored liqueur, but any type will do, and the addition of coffee adds zero calories.

White Wine Spritzer

The concept of the spritzer is simple: white wine mixed in equal proportions with club soda. Depending on the wine you use, this beverage can be refreshingly pleasing and only 100 calories per 5 ounces.

Martini

Martinis are practically straight liquor, but, shaken with ice and an aromatic splash of vermouth, they have a cocktail sensibility and only 160 calories per 2.5 ounces. The strong taste is best suited to someone who likes more flavorful drinks, but infused liquors at a cost of zero extra calories can mellow the flavor.

At no other time should you avoid alcohol more than if you are trying to beat burnout, have a lot to do, or need a clear head. Regardless of how you feel after a couple of drinks, alcohol is a depressant. It will make you tired and groggy but won't necessarily enhance your ability to cope with stress. A few drinks may have you drifting off to sleep, but you could wake up feeling extra tired, queasy, and even more guilty for not accomplishing what you need to get done. Remember: going out and socializing should be about the people, not the alcohol. I believe if you follow these suggestions you'll create positive experiences that you will love remembering the next morning. Balance is beautiful. In moderation, alcohol doesn't have to distract from your health goals. Party smart, keep it classy, and live your life in a healthy, happy way. Always enjoy life. It's happening!

PUTTING IT ALL TOGETHER: HEALTHY EATING FOR LIFE

Why not start today? Clear the junk food out of your cabinets. Take the candy jar off your desk. Remove the temptation, and pick one or two habits to give your diet a healthy boost. Start making changes. The more drastic the change, the higher the possibility for drastic results but also the higher the likelihood that you'll fail as soon as you hit a bump in the road. Balance these changes with your personality. You might stumble a few times before you find your stride or find a method that works for you. Failing or stumbling is okay, as long as you get back up and keep going toward your goals.

Your body wants you to eat well. Eating healthy foods makes you feel better and have more energy, along with reducing digestion problems and mood swings. As you have learned in this chapter, healthy eating doesn't mean *deprivation, tasteless*, or *time-consuming*. It can be delicious, nourishing, and balanced with the foods you love. Eating for energy means eating clean, eating regularly, and eating light. Be moderate with alcohol, stay away from emotional eating, and move more. In a short time your days and nights will not only be filled but fulfilled.

Take action: Pick up your fork and eat something that gives you power.

CHAPTER 4
Rest and Sleep

I know how hard it is to make real time for rest. You feel guilty, like you are wasting time, or think resting is being lazy. Well let me tell you this: if you don't take downtime it will take you down. Rest is a must—it is nonnegotiable! Get in the mind-set that resting isn't cheating, and remind yourself that time off is actually productive. You'll come back from downtime with clarity, purpose, and energy to fuel all your goals. You have to rest if you want to be your best. Here are some life hacks to help you make time for it.

Take 5-minute mini-breaks every hour.
You can't stay focused all the time. No matter how efficiently you work, you'll always get distracted, let your mind wander, or end up reading e-mail and Facebook instead. A better way to spend this time is to get up from your chair, walk outside, and take a 5-minute break. Or stand up and perform a few simple stretches to wake up your body. The change of place,

the change of physical posture, and the movement will make it easier to start again when your break is over. You'll also give your brain a chance to relax and process information, which are essential for your well-being. The human body isn't built to sit in one position for hours while gripping a mouse or typing on a keyboard. Use computer apps like Time Out or your phone alarm to gently remind you to take a break on a regular basis.

Make time for rest.
This is important. Make sure that whenever you plan to rest, you really rest. That means that you will have to make a conscious effort to push away all work-related thoughts and worries. It's also important that you rest your mind as well as your body. For me this means putting away all the electronics. This is a challenge, but unplugging allows for so much peace of mind. Five minutes of real rest is better than 30 minutes in front of the TV.

Take a hot bath with Epsom salts.
Nothing helps me relax more than this kind of bath. Magnesium—the key component of Epsom salt—performs more functions in more systems of the human body than virtually any other mineral, including regulating the activity of more than 325 enzymes. Magnesium is an electrolyte that helps to ensure proper muscle, nerve, and enzyme function. Medical research also indicates that magnesium may reduce inflammation and relieve pain, making it beneficial in the treatment of sore muscles, bronchial asthma, migraine headaches, fibromyalgia, and more. Excess adrenaline and stress are known to drain the body of magnesium, and restoring magnesium levels reduces anxiety, relieves muscle aches, improves sleep, and is as easy as stepping into a hot bath.

To try it, add two cups of Epsom salt to warm water in a standard-size bathtub; double the Epsom salt for an oversized garden tub. Bathe three times weekly, soaking for at least 20 minutes. One hour in the bath may be the best way to relax because of this simple fact: you can't take your work or your computer with you.

Deal with stress with deep breaths, not substances.

It can be tempting to have a drink or eat chocolate to take the edge off a busy, stressful schedule. While a glass of wine or a treat is nice in moderation, using it to cope or numb your stress will eventually sabotage your health long term. Develop a different means of relaxation. Think about other activities that are relaxing and enjoyable to you, like working out, taking a walk outside, listening to music, hanging with a friend, reading, and so on. Schedule those into your life as a means of unwinding. Choose a healthy habit to de-stress with, and you'll actually help yourself.

Get more fresh air and sunlight.

Make sure you get your daily dose of sunlight if you're spending a lot of time inside your home or workplace. Fresh air can be a life changer. Sometimes all you need to do is get outside to shift your mood to a better state.

Take action: Write down three to five healthy habits you feel will help you get quality rest.

Schedule rest time into your day. Personalize your approach to resting/de-stressing. What really works for you and allows you to feel calmer? How can you implement those practices into your lifestyle now for a better state of physical health?

SLEEP YOUR WAY TO THE TOP

When I was in burnout mode, my sleep was poor. I constantly felt tired but wired. I struggled with insomnia and spent many restless nights wishing I could fall asleep. I have so many journal entries from those sleepless nights—pages of anxious words and hope for rest.

When you are overstressed and not taking care of yourself, sleep is usually the first thing to suffer. It then becomes a downward spiral because less sleep equals no energy, mood swings, poor performance, and burnout. Everything starts to shut down when you are trying to be more productive on less sleep, and eventually you self-destruct. The only way to recover from this is to take care of yourself: eat well, exercise, de-stress, take downtime, have some fun. When you aren't mentally or physically healthy, your sleep will suffer. When you aren't getting enough sleep, your mental and physical health will suffer. You need to do both: it goes full circle.

Consistently taking care of your mental and physical fitness will improve your sleep. I promise. There also are a few things you can do right now to improve the quality of your sleep. The first step is to get rid of things in your life that disrupt it. Here are a few things to watch out for or eliminate:

Remove TVs, laptops, tablets, and smart phones from the bedroom.
The LED from these devices is the last thing you need before drifting off to sleep. Remove other sources of bright light, and use soft, warm lighting in your bedroom. Use thick curtains or blinds to remove natural light if you plan to sleep past dawn.

Read your labels on medications and supplements.
If you take medications or supplements, you might be consuming substances that disrupt your sleep without you knowing it. Some supplements contain the stimulants ginseng and
guarana, which have an effect that is similar to caffeine. Some
headache and cold medications also contain caffeine and other
stimulants. Medications such as steroids and beta-blockers can
also keep you awake at night. Check ingredient labels closely,
and talk with your doctor if you suspect that a prescription
medication or supplement is disrupting your sleep.

Say no to the nightcap.
You may feel like a glass of wine or beer makes you feel drowsy,
helping you to sleep better. Well, although it's true that alcoholic drinks may make you drowsy enough to fall asleep
quickly, when your blood alcohol level drops 2 to 3 hours later,
you are likely to wake up. This prevents you from falling into
the deep sleep that helps you wake up feeling rested.

Avoid midnight munchies.
Do your best to avoid late-night snacks and midnight meals.
Late-night eating can negatively affect your digestion and keep
you up past bedtime. If you are hungry late at night, it may
be because you haven't had enough to eat throughout the day,
are bored, are tired, or simply have created a late-night eating
habit. This is a real issue for many people, and staying up late
with food prevents you from living well. Remember: if you are
up late eating, you aren't sleeping—and digesting isn't resting.
Work to undo late-night love affairs with food, and close the
kitchen at a reasonable time so that you can get some quality
rest.

Now lets get you the quality zzz's you need! The following techniques can help you experience deep sleep and start living with more energy. Try one:

Create a Zen sleeping environment.

Your sleep environment is extremely important for sleep quality. Artificial light, warm temperatures, sudden noises, and electromagnetic frequencies (EMFs) can all affect sleep quality, but these things are almost always fixable. Again, you'll have to experiment to figure out what works best for you, but in general it helps to have dark curtains, a soothing setting, fluffy pillows, and calm colors. Aim to keep the temperature between 65 and 68 degrees and always below 70 degrees.

Have regular acupuncture treatments. (It really works. I swear by it.)

Take a hot shower or an Epsom salt bath. (For your convenience, I repeat the details here.)

The magnesium in Epsom salts has been proven to soothe sore muscles and promote deep relaxation. For a salt bath, simply add 2 cups of Epsom salt to warm water in a standard-size bathtub. Bathe three times weekly, soaking for at least 20 minutes. This will help ease muscle pain, fade bruises, flush toxins, and improve sleep.

Exercise regularly.

Doing so will help improve your sleep quality. However, if you are sensitive to stimulation, exercise in the morning or afternoon (not the evening) to allow your body time to come down from the endorphin energy rush long before you prepare for sleep.

Define a sleep bedtime and honor it.

Set a time to go to sleep—and commit to it. When I'm tempted to work later than I should on a project, I kindly remind myself that my "beauty sleep" is the secret to successful work performance.

Leave the computer, tablet, and smart phone out of your bedroom.

Have a "bedtime" for your tech. Being online is overstimulating for your brain. Aim for no Facebook, texts, Tweets, e-mails, or web surfing for at least 30 to 60 minutes before you want to go to sleep.

Foam-roll tight muscles.

A little self-massage can be meditative, help ease tension from the day, and prepare you for a good night's rest.

Stretch or follow a restorative yoga video (there are lots of free, helpful stretch videos on my YouTube channel.)

Journal.

It doesn't have to be an essay. Simply write down a few things you are grateful for or proud of accomplishing so you end the day on a high note.

Have a brain dump.

Take a piece of paper and write down *any* thoughts that are on your mind before bed. To-do lists, ideas, reminders—just put it all on paper so you can rest knowing that it will still be there tomorrow.

Take a magnesium supplement (400–600 milligrams) 30 to 60 minutes before bedtime.

Magnesium is a mineral that's crucial to the body's function. Magnesium helps keep blood pressure normal, bones strong, and the heart rhythm steady. Many people take magnesium as a natural remedy to relieve insomnia. You can also get magnesium from food. Good sources include green leafy vegetables, wheat germ, pumpkin seeds, and almonds. Check with your doctor before taking magnesium supplements.

Avoid caffeine after noon.

Visit your doctor and have your adrenal glands and hormone levels checked.

For both men and women, changes in hormone levels can affect sleep. Hormones change with age and can get out of whack when you're stressed, tired, or eating poorly. When your hormones are imbalanced, it creates all kinds of havoc. Understanding the connections between hormones and sleep may help improve your own sleep and well-being.

Listen to a relaxation CD.

Meditate.

Use the easy and effective Headspace App or try out some free meditations on YouTube.

Read. (I'm all about it!)

Drink chamomile and lime blossom tea before sleeping.

Try some white noise like sounds of rain, ocean, and such, or use a fan to whir you to sleep.

Try sleep affirmations.
Affirmations are simple statements you say to yourself that help to insert positive ideas and suggestions into your brain where they can be surprisingly effective. It is a form of constructive self-talk. Repeat statements such as "My body gets the rest it needs," "I fall to sleep easily and deeply," "I am relaxed and peaceful."

Put lavender on your pillows

Invest in a good mattress.
(You spend one-third of your life sleeping—a good mattress is worth the investment!)

Take extra time for self-care at the end of the day.
Brush your hair, wash and moisturize your face, floss and brush and rinse with mouthwash, stretch, foam-roll. Do whatever it is that makes you feel clean, fresh, and relaxed.

PUTTING IT ALL TOGETHER: GET MORE SLEEP

While all the preceding tips are great, they will only work for you if you make a habit out of them. Create a sleep routine for yourself. We are creatures of habit, and behavior—not just environmental, external cues—helps set our body's rhythms. Put together a pre-sleep ritual that you try to stick to every day. Maybe it's turning off the lights at 9:00 p.m. and switching to candles, followed by a cup of herbal tea, a quick foam roll self-massage, and a good book before bed. Create some standard rituals that you do every night to prepare your body for sleep and that act as cues to your circadian clock to slow down and get ready for bed. Remember: lack of sleep causes stress on the body, weight gain, premature aging, hair loss, hormone imbalances, infertility, lowered immune function, and more burnout. Make yourself a sleep habit, and commit to it. Your body and life will thank you for it.

Take action: Create a soothing sleep environment. How many hours of sleep do you currently get? What's the number that allows you to feel your best? Wind down 30 minutes prior to goal bedtime—no electronics, bright lights, or stimulating music. Put yourself to bed when you need to, and remember the big picture: you can sleep your way to increased productivity, smarter decision making, and more happiness.

CHAPTER 5
Time Management

People always say, "I'm too busy to exercise," "I have to be there for the kids," "I've got too much work." You know what? These are little lies you're telling yourself, and they go against the laws of self-preservation, because the more whole and healthy you are, the more fully you can give to other people.
—Oprah

Our health is one of the most important things we can prioritize, yet it often remains one of the most neglected parts of our busy lives. We all want to eat well, exercise, and take downtime every day. But when everything is moving fast, the world is screaming for your attention, and you just don't have time, the last thing you feel you can do is take time for yourself. Here's the truth, though: the only way you can operate at full speed without crashing is by making your health your number-one priority.

When it comes to being healthy and balanced, time management is everything. Life is a constant juggling act of personal and professional priorities. You want to learn the skills to adapt to life's changes and challenges without running yourself into the ground. The key to juggling is to keep everything in perspective and focus on what's most important to you. When you have a big picture of what you want, then you can use your energy for what's most helpful in making that happen. Chapter 1 allowed you to craft a clear vision of where you want to be. Do your current commitments enable you to move forward toward this big picture? If not, it's time to reprioritize and say no to anything that is keeping you in a state of burnout. It's about learning to make your time work for you so you can realize your wellness vision and create the life you want. Here are some suggestions for how you can manage your time well and move forward toward your big picture.

PUT YOURSELF ON THE CALENDAR

Block out time on your calendar every week for your self-care. Include times for exercise, grocery shopping, meals, pampering yourself, date night, and other self-care. Make this time nonnegotiable time expressly for you. If a potential conflict comes up, try saying something like "I'm so sorry, but I have plans," or "Thanks for thinking of me! I'd love to another time." Allow your self-care time to take precedence over all but real emergencies or important life events, like weddings, funerals, and anniversaries. If you must make a change, reschedule your self-care time for another day that week and stick to it. Treat your self-care appointments like any other essential appointments you can't miss. I have a self-care night every week, during which I read, rest, and unplug from all technology. I book it in advance and look forward to it! My friends and family know when it's self-care night, and I'll be open for business with bright eyes the next day.

> *Take action: Take out your calendar and schedule your self-care. Start with workouts. When will you be working out? For how long? What will you be doing? Next, plan your meals—in writing. When you will go grocery shopping? When would you like to plan to go out to eat with friends? What do you need to have prepared and ready for breakfast, lunch, dinner, and snacks? On what days can you schedule meal prep to save time later in the week?*

Be sure to schedule time for rest. What do you want to do for yourself and when? What do you need to recharge? Whether it's getting a manicure, having time to read, or catching up with a friend over tea, put your downtime into your calendar.

HIRE A PROFESSIONAL

Book an appointment with a coach/trainer/expert. No one is an island—we can't do everything alone. Investing in yourself by getting support from a professional has a huge impact on the degree of your success. You'll have someone working with you to keep you accountable, help you reach your goals, and give you the encouragement you need to stick with taking care of yourself even when life gets hard.

> *Take action: Do a little research on professionals who might be a good fit to work with you. Ask friends for*

their recommendations, or use yelp.com to get some insight on professionals in your area. Start reaching out to people you might like to hire and inquire about their services, rates, and how they work with clients.

What are the results you need and want from working with someone? What is your budget, and how often would you like to work with someone? Are they the right fit, and will they help you accomplish the results you want? Ask potential partners as many questions as you can. Trust your gut on this one: If it feels like the right fit, go for it. If not, keep searching. There is a professional out there who is the perfect fit for you.

CREATE HEALTHY ROUTINES AND PLANS

Fail to plan, and you plan to fail.
—Benjamin Franklin

Thinking ahead is everything when it comes to being successful, and creating healthy habits or routines can make staying on track more effortless. Personalize your approach and find ways to create little habits that help you reach your goals. Everybody is different. Maybe you make it a habit to cook and prep your meals for the week on Sundays. Or you plan ahead for your workouts and prepack clothes in your work bag. Look back on your well-being vision from chapter 1. What are some simple life hacks you could use to cut time, thinking, and effort out of following through with your desired healthy habits? Being organized and establishing healthy routines will allow you more time and space to breathe. Plus the less thinking you have to do, the easier it is to follow through. Set yourself up for success by planning ahead.

Take action: Write down three healthy habits or life hacks that will help you achieve your goals.

Here are some examples of healthy life hacks that can give you more time:

- Plan meals and prepare healthy food one or two days per week to make eating well convenient.
- Pack gym clothes and a gym bag the night before workouts to make it easier to get to the gym at lunch break.
- Use Sunday morning to schedule the week ahead: meals, workouts, social time, rest.
- Go straight to the gym after work and eliminate 30 minutes of extra commuting time.

JUST SAY NO

Take time to consider your top priorities and responsibilities. Do you really have to bake cookies for that fund-raiser? Babysit for your sister? Take on that extra project at work? Attend every Facebook event to which you are invited? Be part of every charity group or recreational sport? Remember that there's nothing wrong with saying no. Yes, we all have commitments to others, but don't forget about the commitments you make to yourself. When you say no to something you can say yes to yourself.

Take action: Write down three little things you can take off your plate to make room for you. What do you want to say no to? What takes up your time and energy? What are the commitments you dread or that drain your energy? What would you like to say yes to instead?

USE THE RIGHT TOOLS

Having the right tools can improve your level of productivity and maximize efficiency. There are so many great resources you can use to keep track of your agenda, manage your time, and increase your productivity. Better time management equals less stress and more success. The following are my favorite time management tools. Check them out!

Time Management and Productivity Tools

Rescuetime
If you have doubts that you are using your time wisely, this app will send you weekly reports to indicate your time thieves. You may be shocked to discover how much time you are wasting. (rescuetime.com)

Remember The Milk
Manage all your tasks effectively. If you are struggling to manage everything you have to do and you work with many different devices, this app is for you. It is a great free tool that is compatible with your mobile devices, computers, Gmail, Outlook, and more. It helps you to manage your tasks easily and reminds you of them wherever you are. (rememberthemilk.com)

SelfControl
Spending more time scrolling through Facebook than working on that looming project? Designed for Mac users, SelfControl gives you a little boost in the productivity department. While you won't be totally unplugging, this app does let you ditch unnecessary distractions. With a blacklist of prohibited sites and a timer (which doesn't run out, even if you restart your

computer), this program makes it easy to avoid clickbait (or your ex-boyfriend's sister's new Facebook album) when you've got more important things on your plate. (selfcontrolapp.com)

Evernote
Capture everything in one place. Evernote is a free productivity tool that allows you to capture all your ideas, thoughts, and images in many different ways, such as with voice, notes, or images. You can record your meetings, interviews, speeches, and ideas and create lists, add voice or text attachments, and share your files with friends. Now you can also sync Remember The Milk with Evernote to really optimize your time. (evernote.com)

focus booster
Need to get something done? This app is based on the principles of the Pomodoro Technique for individuals who procrastinate and feel overwhelmed by tasks. It is designed to empower you to maintain your focus, manage distractions, and get more done. (focusboosterapp.com)

Toggl
Track time spent on projects. This is a great alternative to time sheets if you need to track how much time you spend on different projects. Effective time management starts with knowing exactly how much time you actually spend on your projects and tasks, and then analyzing how you can manage them more effectively. (toggl.com)

Mind42
Put your focus on the tasks at hand. Mind mapping is a great productivity technique, and Mind42 is the best free mind mapping app. It helps you to get more organized by focusing your

thoughts, thereby helping you gain clarity on what you need to do. (mind42.com)

SyncBackFree
Want to back up and sync your files effortlessly? This free software allows you to back up, restore, and synchronize your files easily. It saves you time now as well as in the future. If you have never backed up your files before, you should certainly not overlook this pivotal tool. (2brightsparks.com/freeware)

MyLifeOrganized
Check this out if you find it difficult to manage all your tasks, work with your to-do lists, and organize your goals. This task management system helps you to target what you should be focusing on to reach your objectives. It automatically generates to-do lists, with priority actions for your immediate attention so that you can track your progress methodically. (mylifeorganized.net)

Universal Password Manager
Do you waste time managing all the passwords you have? This app allows you to keep all your passwords in one encrypted database, protected by one password. This saves you time when you forget your passwords and need to retrieve them, and it also allows you to use various passwords so you don't compromise on security. (upm.sourceforge.net)

Tiny Calendar
Do you need to synchronize and access your agenda from different devices? This amazing app syncs all your calendars to give you an instant overview of your day, a calculation of how much time you have until your next meeting, and a

list of your upcoming meetings. (itunes.apple.com/us/app/ tiny-calendar-sync-google)

Pocket
Remove distractions When you are surfing the web, it is so easy to get distracted by enticing websites. Use this tool to save your finds to access and read later at a convenient time that will not impact your work. (getpocket.com)

Focus@Will
Increase your attention span. This amazing app combines neuroscience and music to boost your productivity. It is possible to increase your attention span by up to 400 percent! It's ideal for those who find it difficult to focus while studying, working, or reading. (www.focusatwill.com)

Launchy
Work smarter. This small and simple tool allows you to launch your documents, project files, folders, and bookmarks with just a few keystrokes. This makes life so much easier since you don't need to go through the start menu to access what you want. (www.launchy.net)

So much of burnout comes from feeling overwhelmed by responsibilities, commitments, and to-do lists. But with strong time management skills and the ability to say no, you'll be able to overcome much of that stress. Changing the way you work with time may be the key that unlocks your ability to thrive.

Work smarter, not harder.
—Allan F. Mogensen

PUTTING IT ALL TOGETHER: BALANCED BODY

Congratulations! Now you are on target! The key to maintaining all the positive habits you've now learned is to keep living them every day. Staying on track and staying committed to your decision to eat healthy, exercise regularly, and think positively should now be a habit for life. The whole point of the balanced body program is to introduce you to some simple strategies that can be incorporated into your lifestyle.

If you ever feel overwhelmed by all the information shared in this book, pause and take a deep breath. Remember: you never have to take on more than you can handle, and you can use the suggestions I offer by making them work for you. Take it one step at a time. Progress is progress—no matter how small. Keep moving, be positive, and be proud. Each day you practice your new habits will make you healthier, happier, stronger, and more energetic. Confidence in yourself and your abilities will do more to help you achieve balance than any diet program ever will.

You are a unique, powerful, and rare individual—the one and only you! Taking care of yourself regularly takes courage, consistency, and work, but the payoff is in the quality of your life. Small changes net big results, and any time you invest in feeling your best will pay you back in health.

Remember how lucky you are to be healthy, to have a beautiful body to enjoy. Your health is the greatest gift, and taking care of it allows you to live your life to the max. Give a gift to yourself, your family, and your work by opening up to a happier, healthier, more effective self. Take time to take care of you and enjoy the life you have been given. Make the choice to feel good about yourself, about your world, about your possibilities and the steps you're taking right now. Do so, and you'll be smiling all along the way.

PART III
Balanced Mind

When you are struggling with burnout, it can feel impossible to maintain a positive mind-set. In fact, when you hear people tell you "Just cheer up!" or "Look at the bright side!" you may feel angry or upset. "Easy for them to say," you might think. "Don't they know how much I'm dealing with? How am I supposed to 'look on the bright side' when I'm so stressed out?"

When you are exhausted and overwhelmed it can be difficult to find the energy to be positive. I get that. But you can't live a positive life without having a positive mind first. You'll never leave a state of burnout until you are mentally ready to do it.

When we think about taking care of our health, we think about nutrient-dense foods, exercise, and sleep. But there is something deeper, that is essential to living a balanced life. Just as important as nurturing our physical well-being are the care and feeding of our minds. Studies have shown that 75 to 95 percent of the illnesses that plague us today are a direct result of our thoughts. We know that what we think about affects us physically and emotionally and that the average person has more than 30,000 thoughts a day. If most of those 30,000 daily thoughts are negative, anxious, or fearful, that's like eating poison!

Research shows that fear, all on its own, triggers more than 1,400 known physical and chemical responses and activates more than 30 different hormones. Toxic waste generated by toxic thoughts can cause the following illnesses: diabetes, cancer, asthma, skin problems, and allergies, to name just a few. You know it's true: negative self-talk is limiting, crippling, and harmful. If your words and thoughts carry toxic energies of fear, shame, criticism, judgment, fear, blame, and doubt, you feel depressed, depleted, and dispirited and, well, not in love with your life.

Your mental state has the ultimate influence over how you interact with yourself, with others, and with your world. I can always tell when I'm feeling mentally run down. I feel overly sensitive or struggle with negative thoughts and feelings. I get too caught up in superficial nonsense. I waste time comparing, worrying, or beating myself up. I start to believe my happiness is dependent on the next good thing that may or may not come my way. I have a hard time focusing on all the good and I struggle with a narrow, negative mind.

On the other hand, when I take time to nurture my mental health, I am positive, present, grounded, and at ease. I am comfortable with myself and have strong boundaries that help me maintain balance. I don't take things personally, and I have a clear sense of what really matters to me. I don't sweat the small stuff and am full of energy for my life.

Can you relate? We all can. We are human! Our emotional and mental selves need nurturing and input; they need a focus just like our physical selves do. Your body responds to the way you think, feel, and act; that is the mind/body connection. When you are stressed, anxious, or upset, your body tries to tell you that something isn't right. For example, high blood pressure or a stomach ulcer might develop after a particularly stressful event, such as a fight with a loved one or a big work deadline.

The following can be physical signs that your emotional health is out of balance:

- Back pain
- Change in appetite
- Chest pain
- Constipation or diarrhea
- Dry mouth
- Extreme tiredness
- General aches and pains
- Headaches
- High blood pressure
- Insomnia
- Lightheadedness
- Heart palpitations
- Sexual problems
- Shortness of breath
- Stiff neck
- Sweating
- Upset stomach
- Weight gain or loss
- Frequent colds or infections
- Generally weak immune system

When you are feeling stressed, anxious, or upset, you may not feel like exercising, eating nutritious foods, or socializing with others. Abuse of alcohol, tobacco, or other drugs may also signal poor emotional health. That's why it's important to look after your mind, not just your body. It really is what's on the inside that counts.

So, which comes first: the physical or the mental fitness? Both. Getting your body in a balanced state of health will help you train a positive mind, and a positive mind will help you achieve a balanced, healthy body. You'll see both mind and body start to improve as you continue to take action toward taking care of yourself, beating burnout, and achieving your vision of success.

The number-one thing I see holding people back from moving forward toward a strong mind-set is that they are focused on the wrong things. They are thinking about past mistakes, living in a language of "can't," and obsessed with everything that's going wrong in their life. Here's something you need to understand: what you focus on expands. That's why when you focus on how stressed you are and how many problems you have, you'll only find more stress and problems.

We think too much about what goes wrong and not enough about what goes right in our lives. Of course, sometimes it makes sense to analyze bad events so that we can learn from them and avoid them in the future. However, we tend to spend more time thinking about what is bad in life than what is good. Worse, this focus on negative events sets us up for anxiety, depression, and even more burnout. One way to keep this from happening is to get better at thinking about and savoring everything that's going well. In the chapters in this part of the book, you will learn how to use the positive thought diet, positive affirmations, gratitude, and stress management techniques. These tools will allow you to focus on the positive so that you can bring more positive into your life. We then will work together to create your mental workout plan, so that you can train positively and leave burnout behind.

CHAPTER 6

The Positive Thought Diet

Burnout comes with mental and emotional exhaustion. Constant fatigue causes you to feel trapped, defeated, unmotivated, cynical, and/or negative. This mental funk keeps you stuck, and disables you from taking positive steps forward to work your way into a better state. You will never leave burnout without the right thoughts to help you.

It has been said that the only true disability in life is a negative attitude. I believe that's true and that positive thinking enables you to do everything better. It also helps with stress management and even can improve your health. Researchers continue to explore the effects of positive thinking and optimism on well-being. Health benefits may include any or all of these:

- Increased life span
- Lower rates of depression
- Lower levels of distress

- Greater resistance to the common cold
- Better psychological and physical well-being
- Reduced risk of death from cardiovascular disease
- Better coping skills during hardships and times of stress

Positive thinking isn't about ignoring problems but, rather, about overcoming them. It often starts with self-talk, the endless stream of unspoken thoughts that run through your head every day. These automatic thoughts can be positive or negative. If they are mostly negative, your outlook on life is more likely pessimistic. If they are mostly positive, you're likely an optimist—someone who practices positive thinking.

Have you been having too many negative thoughts lately? Are they causing you to feel defeated, tired, stressed, upset, unhappy? Are they creating adverse reactions like overeating, random acts of anger, apathy, sleeplessness, or lack of interest in your life? Why do you keep allowing them if they make you feel sick?

You can learn to turn negative thinking into positive thinking. It takes time and practice to create this new habit. However, if you follow my positive thought diet, you will start to think and behave in a more positive and optimistic way.

I believe the only diet you ever really need to be on is a positive thought diet: detox your mind from thoughts that make you feel sick and take away your ability to fully enjoy your life. Take out the trash talk, and your life will eventually get cleaned up the way you want. No one is perfect; we all struggle with this. But simply building an awareness over the thoughts that control your life can help you be more in control of the thoughts you choose to cultivate. You mind is a garden, and your thoughts are the seeds. You can grow flowers, or you can grow weeds. Want to get rid of the weeds and grow flowers instead? Get on the positive thought diet—110 percent results guaranteed. Here's how:

Clean out the criticism cabinet.

Look in your mental cabinet and clean out all criticism. Criticism never changes a thing. Refuse to criticize yourself. Accept yourself exactly as you are, and encourage yourself to grow with positive self-talk. Everybody changes. When you criticize yourself, your changes are negative. When you approve of yourself, your changes are positive.

Feed yourself forgiveness on a weekly basis.

Let the past go. You did the best you could at the time with the understanding, awareness, and knowledge that you had. Now you are growing and changing, and you will live life differently. It's a process. Forgive regularly and keep moving forward.

Don't believe scary, false packaging.

Stop scaring yourself with fearful, terrorizing thoughts. It's an awful way to live. Remember that FEAR stands for FALSE EVIDENCE APPEARING REAL. Don't waste your life hanging out with your fearful thoughts. Acknowledge them and call them out. Face your fears and they disappear.

Marinate the mind with positive juices.

Our mind is a sponge. It absorbs almost everything it encounters. From the negative comment a work colleague made a year ago to some awful things heard on the news, we can't but help internalize all the things our senses pick up. Sadly there is a lot of negativity in the world. Positive thinking isn't about ignoring the negative—it's about overcoming it. To do this, you must marinate the mind with positive influences on a daily basis. From surrounding yourself with positive people, reading inspirational blogs, or watching TED talks, do what it takes to be more proactive about what you put into your mind rather than just allowing others to influence it. Regularly feeding positive things (words, messages, conversations, stories, pictures, etc.) to your mind will help you overcome the negative influences of the world with optimism.

Take daily doses of gentleness morning, noon, and night.
Be gentle with yourself. Be kind to yourself. Be patient with yourself as you learn how to follow the positive diet and think new ways of thinking. Treat yourself as you would someone you really loved. Feed yourself with compassion and care regularly throughout your day.

Be kind to your mind at all times.
Self-hatred is merely hating your own thoughts. Don't hate yourself for having the thoughts. We are all human—we all struggle with this. Gently work to change your thoughts and be kind to yourself in the process.

Praise yourself.
Criticism breaks down the inner spirit. Praise builds it up. Praise yourself as much as you can. Tell yourself how well you are doing with every little thing. Celebrate your progress.

Serve yourself with support.
Find ways to support yourself at every opportunity. Reach out to friends and allow them to help you. Set boundaries and honor your commitments to yourself. Being strong means practicing self-care, asking for help when you need it, and finding ways to support yourself toward living the life you want.

Learn everything you can about positive life fueling.
Don't let the positive diet be a quick fix or fad in your life. Learn everything you can about living your best life and keep learning. Learn about nutrition. What kind of fuel does your body need in order to have optimum energy and vitality? Learn about exercise. What kind of exercise do you enjoy? Learn about self-care. What do you need to feel balanced and well? Cherish and revere the body and soul you were blessed to live in—and never stop.

Sip on self-love 24/7.
Don't wait until you get well, or lose the weight, or get the new job, or find the new relationship. Begin now—and do the best you can. I have found that one thing heals every problem and that is to love yourself. When people start to love themselves more each day, it's amazing how their lives get better. They feel better. They get the jobs they want. They have the money they need. Either their relationships improve or the negative ones dissolve and new ones begin. Loving yourself is a lifetime of learning and practice: you get better at it, but you never stop practicing. Just like a muscle that you work out in the gym, if you don't use it you will lose it. And just like drinking water, self-love is key for flourishing in life. Start now. Drink it up!

Happiness and health are an inside-out process, and I believe that by following the positive thought diet you will think well, live well, and be well in your life. Watch the thoughts you are feeding yourself. You can't live a happy, healthy life with an unhappy, unhealthy mind. Are you ready to work on feeding yourself more positive thoughts? Let's work out the mind with positive affirmations or, as I like to call them, "mental push-ups"!

MENTAL PUSH-UPS: THE POWER OF
POSITIVE AFFIRMATIONS

When I was recovering from burnout, I used positive self-talk to keep my mind focused on the wellness vision I wanted to accomplish. Inspired by my goals, I developed a positive affirmation I would repeat over and over to myself: "Strong, confident, vibrant, and full of energy. I make great money helping people realize their goals and dreams."

According to my friends at Lululemon, the mind can only hold one thought at a time. I figured if that was true and my mind was focused on my positive self-statement instead of all the stress from my burnout, it would help. Guess what? It worked.

I learned firsthand that, when used properly, positive self-talk and affirmations can turn your life around. Sound too airy-fairy for you? I want you to give it a real, heartfelt try and see what results you experience. Your equation for success is as follows:

Positive Thoughts = Positive Actions = Positive Results

It has been said that performance is 90 percent perception and 10 percent reality. Each of us is constantly engaging in our own internal thought processing. We talk to ourselves and interpret our situations based on our own perceptions of what is going on around us. If our self-talk is positive, then we function quite well, take positive actions, and move forward. If our thoughts are irrational, exaggerated, or negative, then we may become anxious or emotional and our performance is likely to decline. The words you use to talk to yourself have tremendous power over your mind, body, performance, and results. That's why it is critical to become aware of what thoughts and self-statements are running your actions and ultimately your life.

What Is an Affirmation?

An affirmation is a strong, positive self-statement, spoken in the present tense about a goal that has the potential for being accomplished. It is a preplanned statement of an aspiration, presented to the mind as if it has already been achieved. You present it to the mind in the present tense rather than the future tense. Although intellectually you know your goal is in the future, successful mental programming dictates that it be stated in the present tense as an already realized fact. The mind and the body are so well connected that the body often doesn't know whether a phrase or image is real, dreamed, or imagined. So when your mind creates an image of success, your central nervous system and whole body will process that image as if it were real. Most of the time our actions are reflections of our mental pictures. Which means that choosing the right words and thoughts can make or break our performance.

Affirmations are a powerful way to cancel or correct long-standing negative thoughts or ideas that might be keeping you stuck in burnout. A positive affirmation helps create an attitude or posture in life that says "I can do this!" It is a conscious, carefully worded positive statement that guides your behaviors in a constructive way. It empowers you to replace pessimistic scripts with new creative phrases to help you move forward. These words then become effective tools for transforming your perception of daily events and in turn your actions toward positive results.

I often use affirmations with my coaching clients to help them reconstruct their thoughts to be more positive. I encourage people to use empowering self-statements like "I am healthy, strong, fit, and full of energy" or to repeat a mantra such as "strong, focused, motivated, dedicated." These mantras or affirmations aid in overcoming mental obstacles and accomplishing goals with power.

You can maximize your chances of getting the results you want and create real changes in your life by using affirmations. Use affirmations to achieve the following:

- Improve concentration
- Relax and sleep well
- Build self-confidence
- Accelerate learning
- Deal with fear and negativity
- Heal quickly from sickness or injury
- Increase endurance, strength, and performance
- Train faster and more efficiently
- Improve relationships
- Improve quality of life and well-being

The subconscious mind is literal and factual in nature, just like the hard drive of a computer. It receives information exactly the way you present it. That's why when using affirmations it's important not to use statements that are negative like "I hope I don't stress out over this work project" and instead to use statements in the positive like "I have worked hard and am well prepared for this work project." Affirmations must be presented in a specific way to optimize their effectiveness.

Using Affirmations for a
Balanced Body Breakthrough

Here are my guidelines for creating affirmations that work.

Use the present tense.
Act as if it is already happening. Instead of "I want to be fit," use "I am healthy, strong, and fit."

Use a positive outlook.
When you use negative words, they may be taken into your brain without your awareness. Negative thoughts are like affirmations for what you *don't* want. Affirm what you *do* want to have happen instead. Rather than saying "I will not eat so much junk food," say "I choose to eat well and nourish my body."

Use self-image statements.
When possible, construct your affirmations beginning with "I" or "I am" or "I enjoy" or "I choose."

Keep your affirmation short, clear, and specific.
Make your affirmations a clear statement of your feelings. This way you can easily remember the phrase and your mind can take it in.

Make your affirmations permanent.
"I am strong, vibrant, and healthy!" "I love exercising in the mornings." "When I feel good, I exercise. When I exercise, I feel good." "I am balanced and well."

Use mood words.
Include words that suggest strong, positive emotions. "I am full of energy and positivity." "I always get excited for workouts."

Anticipate success.
When creating your affirmations, don't let your critical side limit the phrases you create. Use whatever thoughts work for you and inspire you.

Use cards, sticky notes, smartphones, vision boards, text reminders—whatever works!
Write your affirmations on something you will look at often. Your computer desktop, fridge magnet, car dashboard, or bathroom mirror—anything works if it works for you. I have my affirmations on my smartphone alarm clock. When I turn off my daily morning alarm, I see phrases like "Today is going to ROCK!"

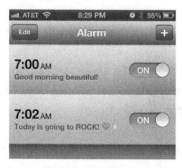

Here are a few samples of health and fitness affirmations to get you started:

♥ I am healthy, happy, and radiant.
♥ I appreciate and love my body.
♥ I love feeling fit and strong. It is easy for me to eat well and exercise regularly.
♥ The older I get, the healthier I become.
♥ I radiate good health.
♥ I am calm and at peace.
♥ I am focused and motivated.

♥   My sleep is relaxed and refreshing.

♥   I have all the energy I need to accomplish my goals.

♥   My body is healed, restored, and filled with energy.

♥   I have abundant energy, vitality, and well-being.

♥   My body maintains its ideal weight and health.

♥   I am filled with energy for all the daily activities in my life.

♥   My mind is at peace.

♥   I choose to be at a healthy weight.

♥   Every day, in every way, I am becoming better and better.

♥   I am healthy and happy.

♥   I love and care for my body, and it cares for me.

PUTTING IT ALL TOGETHER: TRAINING A POSITIVE MIND

You will want to attach positive emotions to your affirmations. Think about how achieving your goal will make you feel, or think about how good it feels to know that you are good at something. Emotion is a fuel that makes affirmations more powerful. If you find yourself simply reciting the words of your affirmations, instead of concentrating on their meaning, change your affirmations. You can still affirm the same goals or characteristics, of course, but rephrasing your affirmations can rejuvenate their effectiveness. Don't be discouraged if your affirmations don't seem to help at first. Instead, think about how you are using them. Do you really believe them? If you don't believe the affirmations, they can still be effective, but it will take longer.

When you use affirmations to counteract negative scripts or to accomplish small goals, you will eventually develop the confidence to tackle bigger issues. Your goal should be to repeat your affirmation daily and often—morning, noon, night, and in-between. Repetition builds belief, and positive belief builds success.

It's important to keep experimenting with new ways of thinking until you find what is right for you. Next time you are upset, listen to the words you use with yourself. Notice if they are reinforcing worn-out ways of thinking or encouraging a fresh outlook. Try to choose words that invite constructive changes.

Work against the negative thoughts related to burnout by strengthening your mind by using the positive thought diet and positive affirmations. Remember that affirmations are like mental push-ups: do enough of them, and your mind will get positively buff.

When you change the way you talk to yourself, you feel happier, stronger, and healthier as a result. I've said it a million times and I'll say it again: positive thoughts = positive actions = positive results!

CHAPTER 7

Gratitude Is a Game Changer

In daily life we must see that it is not happiness that makes us grateful. But gratefulness that makes us happy.
—*Brother David Steindl-Rast*

When I was struggling with burnout, gratitude was a game changer that turned my world around. I was stuck in a negative, exhausted funk and I didn't know how to climb out of it. My mother (the most positive woman I know) suggested I start keeping gratitude journal. I was desperate for a tool to turn my life around and so I picked up a pen and started writing. I choose to journal three things each day that I was thankful for. Every day may not be good, but there's something good in every day. It wasn't always easy, but I was determined to celebrate the blessings in my life instead of the challenges. And then miracles started to happen because by focusing on the positive I found even more to be thankful for.

Practicing gratitude can center you, help you live in the moment, enhance your relationships, empower you to overcome hurdles, improve your health, and motivate you to reach your goals. When you think about it, reaching any goal starts with a single positive thought. Feeling grateful for what you have can produce the good feelings that keep you moving toward the happy life you want. It is not happy people who are thankful; it is thankful people who are happy.

If you are struggling with burnout, you might feel trapped in a pattern of negative thinking. It only takes one negative thought to breed more, and before you know it you're even more stressed, unhappy, and frustrated. Negative thinking is a sinking ship; once you are in it, it's hard to get out of it. This downward spiral can eventually create other ailments in your life, including constant fatigue, depression, and isolation (because really, who wants to hang out with a negative person?). Believe it or not, you can use gratitude as a tool to reprogram your thoughts, break out of a negative funk, and generate more happiness in your life. The best way to do this is by starting a daily gratitude practice.

If you spend a few minutes every day reflecting on what you're grateful for I can pretty much guarantee you'll see a snowball effect, resulting in physical, psychological, and social benefits. One study published in the *Journal of Psychosomatic Research* confirmed that individuals who had a more grateful outlook got better quality shut-eye, stayed asleep longer, and required less time to fall asleep than their less grateful peers. Perhaps more impressive, people who spent time focusing on grateful thoughts exercised for 1.5 more hours each week, compared to people who spent time focusing on the hassles in their life, according to a study in the *Journal of Personality and Social Psychology*. And at least eight studies have shown that people who express gratitude tend to show fewer symptoms of depression.

HOW TO START A GRATITUDE PRACTICE

Keep a gratitude journal.
Studies show that people who make weekly gratitude journal entries feel better about their lives and more optimistic about the future. Not into breaking out the pen and paper? Try using a smartphone app. I like the Five Minute Journal iOS app, which prompts users each day to write down three things they're grateful for, three things that would make the day awesome, and three affirmations, such as "I am confident" or "I am kind."

Write a letter to someone who left a mark.
Remember that teacher or professor who helped you explore your passions? Or the mentor who gave you the confidence to ace that presentation? Grab some stationery and write out a handwritten thank you. You'll benefit from the pleasant memories of positive events and people in your life. Plus, your recipient will feel pretty great reading about your fond memories of them.

Give a genuine compliment to someone.
Make someone else's day and give them a genuine compliment. Tell someone he or she looks awesome, did a great job, or rocked a workout. They'll feel like a million bucks—quite literally, since receiving a compliment lights up the same regions of the brain that get activated when you receive an award, studies suggest. This region of the brain controls memory and

learning, and researchers believe compliments can help us perform better for days after being given praise.

Make your gratitude public.

Posting on social media or participating in an online gratitude project can help you pay your grateful feelings forward. According to data scientists at Facebook, emotions are contagious on the social network. Post a grateful status update, and your friends might feel more positive. Don't want to bombard your personal newsfeed every day? At the Gratitude Jar website (http://www.gratitudejar.com), read why other people around the world are feeling grateful, and add your own positive thoughts to the "jar." Or put your blessings on the World Gratitude Map (https://gratitude.crowdmap.com).

Take Instagram photos of things, places, and people who make life joyful and bright.

Work to shift a setback or challenge into something positive or an opportunity to grow and learn something.

PUTTING IT ALL TOGETHER: LIVING IN GRATITUDE

We might not have the power to control everything in our lives, but we do have the power to choose our thoughts and focus them on the positive. Practicing gratitude is one of the best ways to do this, and I've found it helps create the right attitude that can promote change in your life. I've found so much encouragement, happiness, and love from celebrating what I'm grateful for rather than what I don't have. It takes work, but you can learn to focus on gifts in even the most dire situations. Though it may seem difficult and unnatural at first, having a gratitude practice and choosing to focus on the positive every day will help you cultivate a greater sense of happiness and optimism about your life. Gratitude isn't about believing that life is perfect but, rather, identifying happiness when we look at our lives as a whole. Remember: no matter how tired or burned out you feel, there is always, always, always something to be grateful for.

CHAPTER 8

Managing Stress for a Healthier Mind-Set

Whether it's physical, emotional, situational, or a combination of everything, burnout is a result of too much stress. Stress isn't always bad. In small doses, it helps you perform under pressure and motivates you to do your best. Past a certain point, though, it stops being helpful and starts causing major damage to your health, mood, productivity, relationships, and quality of life.

Going nonstop without taking care of yourself is a recipe for disaster. When you're constantly running around in emergency -fight-or flight mode, you continually trigger the stress response and never fully return to a healthy balance. This results in chronic stress that can wreak havoc on nearly every system in your body. It can raise blood pressure, suppress the immune system, increase the risk of heart attack and stroke, contribute to infertility, speed up the aging process, and leave you vulnerable to a bunch of mental and emotional problems.

Life is not meant to be lived as a marathon during which you keep running and running and whoever goes the longest wins. Life is actually a series of sprints. You sprint, sprint, sprint, and then rest and recover. That way you're always exerting maximum effort for the best result, but you rest so you don't burn out. Right now you might feel like you are a hamster on a wheel going round and round, pushing yourself all the time, and this has caused you to break down. In order to be filled with energy, overcome burnout, and live a powerful life, it's important to learn how to take time off. Going the extra mile to help your body regenerate and cope with the hundreds of daily stressors you face has a huge impact.

We often wait until something happens, and then we react. This is why our health sometimes fails, we have meltdowns, and maybe it's the reason you are reading this book right now. We're so busy running that we don't stop until our bodies shut down and force us to take notice of the damage we've done. It's time to take a positive approach and prevent stress from overwhelming your health and your life. Sometimes you have to go slow in order to go fast. By recharging your batteries and taking care of yourself, you will set the foundation that will have you feeling great and living without burnout.

One key to your success lies in having the right resources and strategies to cope with, manage, and overcome stress. To beat burnout and live in balance, your long-term solutions must be realistic and focus on lifestyle changes. In this chapter I help you to identify what triggers your stress and personalize your approach to overcoming it with all-natural strategies that work.

COMMON STRESS TRIGGERS

The first step in developing preventive methods to overcome stress is identifying what triggers it. This means ruling out behavioral factors that may be impacting your stress level. Behavioral factors include excessive caffeine consumption, poor nutrition, drugs, alcohol, and toxic environments, among others. Here I've listed some elements within your control that may adversely affect your stress and ability to climb out of burnout.

Caffeine
Caffeine is a stimulant that can trigger an anxiety attack. It is also extremely acidic, which leads to inflammation (bad for overall health) and a diuretic (contributes to dehydration). Be mindful of your consumption of caffeine; cut back if you need to, and moderate your intake. Four cups of coffee before noon, diet cola with lunch, an afternoon energy drink, and evening tea do not qualify as moderate caffeine consumption.

Alcohol
Alcohol also is acidic and dehydrating. Drinking alcohol can overwork your liver and may interfere with your body's ability to properly use oxygen, which can make you more sensitive to stress. Also, alcohol masks the symptoms of stress and is a form of self-medication that ultimately exacerbates you problems.

Drugs and/or prescription medications
Prescribed or not, drugs can alter your body's functioning and make it difficult to control your moods and emotions. Medications often can cause depression, mood swings, anxiety, and increased vulnerability to stress. Be a conscious consumer. Talk to your doctor if you are taking any prescription

drugs (birth control, allergy medicine, pain medication, supplements, herbs, etc.) that you feel may be adversely affecting you. If you are experiencing mood swings or heightened stress, it may be coming from your medicine.

Dehydration

As mentioned, alcohol and caffeine lead to dehydration, as do processed, sugary foods and a general lack of sufficient H_2O. Dehydration interferes with proper brain and body functioning, which can be a trigger for anxiety and depression. Aim to consume half of your body weight in ounces of water per day. Check out chapter 3 regarding nutrition for my suggestions on hydration.

Sleep deprivation

Lack of sleep can make you more vulnerable to stress by making you edgy, unfocused, and hormonally imbalanced. Between 7 and 8 hours of sleep each night are recommended for your body to renew, restore, and replenish. Make sleep a priority and work toward getting 7 to 8 hours nightly.

Toxic environments

A toxic environment is any situation in which the work, the atmosphere, the people, or any combination of these dismays you so much that it causes serious disruptions elsewhere in your life. Make no mistake: everything can be challenging at times, but you know an environment is toxic when it's draining the life out of you. If you are in a toxic environment, you will begin to see problems with your personal health. If you feel like you are in a situation that is negative, demanding, or unhealthy, you need to ask yourself what your options are. Toxic environments come and go, and if you can learn something from it, great. If you have the ability to leave it and move on to a healthier (nontoxic) environment, do so as soon as possible.

NATURAL WAYS TO EASE STRESS AND BEAT BURNOUT

Stress is part of life, but if you are equipped with the right coping strategies, it doesn't have to lead to burnout. Start by resolving any negative lifestyle factors so that you are not as susceptible to melting under pressure. Then personalize your approach to managing stress through effective, natural, healthy methods. It's about being preventive, proactive, and finding coping techniques that work for you. The following are some of my suggestions for all-natural ways to ease and manage stress.

Exercise

You learned in chapter 2 how powerful exercise can be in coping with stress. Exercise helps flush toxins and lowers anxiety and depression-provoking chemicals and hormones while it increases feel-good hormones. It also fosters deeper sleep, an important piece in managing stress well.

Meditation

You may feel like you are too busy, unable to sit still, or incapable of quieting your mind long enough to meditate. That might be exactly why you need it. Meditation has been proven to reduce stress, improve concentration, increase self-awareness, benefit cardiovascular and immune health, increase happiness, slow aging, and encourage a healthy lifestyle. Meditation doesn't have to be complex or involve special pillows; it can be something as simple as sitting still for several minutes and focusing on your breathing while clearing your mind. There is no right or wrong way to do it. Every good meditation practice must begin with finding what and where work best for you. Here are some effective meditation techniques that can actually help your ever-racing mind to relax.

Guided meditations

Hundreds of resources online contain a huge supply of guided meditations and music to help soothe your soul. Try perusing Google Play, iTunes, or SoundCloud for guided meditations and stress-reducing sounds.

Visualization

Another easy and down-to-earth meditation technique is to picture a peaceful state or setting in your mind. Focus on the picture, and let yourself embellish it as much or as little as you need. Use all your senses and imagine how it would feel, smell, taste, and be to visit your picture. I like to take myself to Hawaii. The fresh scent of plumeria and the sound of waves crashing on the beach instantly put me in relaxation mode.

Mantra meditation

Repeating words over and over again is a meditation technique that can help you find calm and focus. You can choose to use your positive affirmations or one word, such as *peace*, which instantly makes you feel at ease. It doesn't matter what you choose—just that you feel good about your choice.

Present moment meditation

This meditation technique is all about fully experiencing the present moment. Close your eyes and focus on your breath for a few moments. Then allow your focus to broaden to your body and the sensations that it's feeling. Next, expand your focus to anything touching your body, noticing those sensations. Last, expand your awareness to everything you can hear and sense. Now reverse this process and come back, one step at a time, to your breath.

Observe your thoughts meditation
Close your eyes and focus on the spot about an inch above the spot between your eyebrows. Begin to watch what your mind and body are feeling, thinking, and doing. Focus on becoming the observer of your mind.

Moving meditation
You don't have to sit still to find peace of mind. Go for a walk, swim, run, or hike, and make it a meditation by focusing on every piece of the experience (this is similar to the present moment meditation). Watch your breath, notice every step, and be completely in the moment. When you are at one with the present moment, fully experiencing all the sensations, I believe you will also gain the benefits of a sitting still meditation practice.

Self-massage meditation
I find self-massage to be very meditative, and it connects me to my body in a positive way. At night, before I go to sleep, I set a phone alarm for 10 to 20 minutes and foam-roll. It's soothing and deeply relaxing, calming my mind and helping me come down from my day. If you are the type of person who enjoys self-massage like I do, this might be a good technique for you.

Download and say OM

Smartphone apps can help you meditate. Put your smartphone on airplane mode and take some time to unwind with a guided meditation app. My favorite smartphone app suggestions are included at the end of this chapter.

Caroline's "Take a Moment" Meditation

Done regularly with intention, this exercise can change your life.

> *Take a good look at your life right now. If you don't like something about it, close your eyes and imagine the life you want. Now allow yourself to focus your thoughts on the person you would be if you were living this preferred life. Notice the differences in how you behave, present yourself, and feel. Allow yourself to spend several seconds breathing in the new image, expanding your energy into this new mold. Hold the image for several seconds and allow it to imprint on your subconscious mind.*

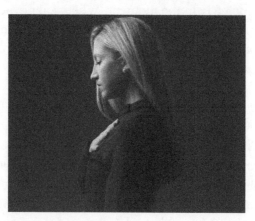

When it feels like you're being pulled in every direction by forces beyond your control, it's time to realign yourself with what you value most in life. The way to do this is to clear the distractions, the outside noise, and the external world, and go inward.

Meditation is an approach to training the mind, similar to the way that fitness is an approach to training the body. Just like fitness, the more you train the mind, the stronger you'll become. So how do you learn to meditate? Practice. Take the preceding suggestions and see what works for you. The goal is to find a regular activity to focus your mind and restore your calm. For best results, start with 10 minutes of meditation. If you can do it daily, great! If not, practice when you can! You might find your racing mind starts to slow down and becomes more powerful, present, and calm.

One of my favorite quotations of Lao Tzu is, "At the center of your being you have the answer. You know who you are and you know what you want." Give yourself time and space to connect to the center of your being, to who you are and what you want. I believe a daily meditation can serve as a simple and powerful way to quiet your mind and direct your life in the direction you want.

Set Boundaries with Technology

I experience higher levels of stress when my boundaries with technology are out of whack. The more plugged in I am, the more anxious I feel. Each ding or buzz makes everything seem urgent. The more addicted I am to tech, the more frazzled and anxious I get. For me, setting limits on my phone, e-mail, texts, and social media offers one of the most effective ways to calm my busy mind and live in health.

Our world is addicted to the cell phone and e-mail. There's a reason the nickname for the Blackberry has become "Crackberry." We are known as the connected generation, and there are obvious issues that have stemmed from our constantly plugged-in state. The Pew Research Center states that Millennials (those who came of age in the new millennium—currently ages 20 to 36) are the "always-on generation." That's absolutely correct. We text and Snapchat and Kik our friends. We Instagram what we eat and post where we are on Facebook—and that's all before lunch. We can't seem to get by without some sort of tech. We are living life through a device, and it's not healthy. If you are feeling burned out or stressed, it could be your overconnectivity to tech. Here are some signs that it might be time for a digital detox.

Signs of an Unhealthy, Stressful Relationship to Technology

- You text and talk at the same time.
  You ask the person in front of you to wait so you can finish a text, watch a video, or read a post, and you rarely notice when they walk off.
- You text and walk (or drive!) at the same time.
  Not only does it take you twice as long to get to your destination, it's *just.not.safe*. If you can't resist commuting while texting, it might be time to turn off your phone. (I like you. Please, no accidents!)
- You feel naked without your phone.
  Have you ever left your phone at home and panicked? That's not a good sign. If you break out in a sweat without your tech, it's a sign you're an addict.
- You repeatedly end up online longer than you originally intended. Are you spending late nights "accidentally" surfing Instagram or Facebook? No wonder you are tired!

- You spend more time with your friends online than you do in the real world.
- You deny it (sometimes defensively) when another person makes a negative comment about how much time you spend online.
- You check your mobile phone in the bathroom. (That's way too common. Ew! Please don't text while you poop!).
- You wait impatiently to get done with real interactions so that you can get online or check your phone.
- You find yourself distracted by thoughts of how many Facebook notifications, e-mails, or texts you might have to reply to.
- You have a hard time maintaining focus on a project, conversation, or event.
- You don't know how to *not* Instagram an experience. You spend an excessive amount of time posting about yourself or absorbed in your phone during friends' outings, events, or vacations.
- You feel a physical and emotional urge to check in with your online community throughout the day.
- You base part of your self-worth on how many followers you have on Twitter, Facebook, or Instagram.
- You never take a break from responding, tweeting, e-mailing, texting, and so on. You live in fight-or-flight mode, and your nervous system is frazzled. You are anxious, stressed, and overtired.

If you related to any of the preceding statements, it may be time to work on a healthier relationship to your tech. Your relationship to tech could be keeping you stuck in a state of burnout. You don't have to live your life through a device. Here are my tips for working with technology to enhance your life instead of allowing your tech to create excessive stress.

Tips for a Healthy Relationship with Tech

Create NO phone and social media time zones.
Set aside times in your day to put the phone away, exit out of all social media, and focus on what you are doing. I hold "office hours" for myself in the morning where I literally put my phone in the closet and close out of all distractions (it's the truth!). This way I'm not tempted to innocently check my notifications during work and can enjoy my morning distraction free and present. Doing one task mindfully does a world of good for my stress and anxiety. I'm a huge advocate for creating no-phone time zones for yourself. This means that for at least a few hours of your day you close off your phone and stay completely dedicated to what's in front of you.

Create a digital bedtime.
Power off your phone and computer an hour before bed to ensure that your last hour is spent in a meaningful way and that you get to sleep on time to start the next day afresh. I like to set a bedtime for my tech and power off at a set time at night. Your tech is not worth losing sleep over. Leave your devices in another room so that you can get the real rest you need without distraction.

Remember that you teach people how to text and e-mail you.
If you respond to texts, e-mails, or phone calls at all hours of the day, people will think you are available at all hours of the day. If you don't want people contacting you at a certain time, DON'T RESPOND DURING THAT TIME. If you don't set boundaries for yourself no one else will.

Manage your time well.
Successful people don't waste hours surfing online and successful people aren't slaves to their e-mail. Lifehack.org offers this observation: "The biggest obstacle to productivity is connectivity." You want to be successful? Manage your time well.

Get real.
When you are with friends and people you care about, commit to being present. Always put the real person before the digital one.

When on a trip, pack your phone in your suitcase or somewhere out of reach for two hours at a time.
Gradually increase the amount of time you disconnect. Enjoy the scenery, the moment, and the people in it. Experience it!

Set a timer for how long you want to spend surfing the web or using your tech.
Set it and stick to the allotted amount of time. That way you can still get your fix without overdoing it.

Take a digital detox weekend or retreat.
Book yourself a holiday and leave all technology at home. If this sounds like a huge challenge, chances are that you need it. Give yourself a break from all tech and come back with a new perspective and feeling refreshed.

Remind yourself that your success and self-worth are not dependent on how many followers you have on Facebook.
You don't need external validation to tell yourself that you are amazing, and you don't need a million followers to live a life you love. Care less about who you are online and more about who you are in your life. You will have fewer disappointments

and more meaningful moments the minute you stop seeking from others the validation only you can give yourself. You are so much more than your clout.

Don't get me wrong—technology's great. But it's supposed to serve us; we're not supposed to be slaves to it. We must learn to unplug from our devices and plug back into our lives in order to truly thrive. To eliminate stress and increase life satisfaction, make it a priority to set boundaries when it comes to technology. Getting past a state of stress or burnout could start with the simple act of unplugging.

Aromatherapy

Inhaling essential oils can alter brain activity. Seek out scents that induce calm, such as lavender, jasmine, rose, and sandal-wood. Use scent as part of a calming ritual, like a warm bath with lavender oil before bed with a cup of chamomile tea. You can also carry a small bottle of essential oil with you to use while taking breathing breaks throughout your day.

Hydration

Dehydration interferes with proper brain and body function-ing, which can be a trigger for anxiety and depression. Aim to consume half of your body weight in ounces of water per day. Foods high in water content also count, so feel free to load up on fruits and veggies. Increasing water intake flushes toxins and other depression-contributing elements from your system at a faster rate and keeps your brain, digestive, and circulatory systems in their prime.

Deep Breathing

The thing people rave about the most at the end of my seminars and workshops are the deep breathing exercises. It always surprises me, out of all the information I present, how powerful the breath work can be. That's because the simple act of breathing does a lot more than move oxygen throughout the body. It stimulates the parasympathetic nervous system, which promotes a state of calm.

Breathing techniques help you connect to your body, shift your awareness away from worries, and quiet your mind. Breathing exercises are free, can be practiced anywhere, and are highly effective in fighting off burnout. Regularly using deep breathing exercises to stay focused, present, and calm will allow you to manage high levels of stress without having a meltdown. The key is finding the breathing techniques that work for you. Here are some simple deep breathing exercises that really work.

Deep belly breathing
This technique is my favorite because it's simple, easy to use, and highly effective. When you are under stress, you often breathe in a shallow manner, not using your full lung capacity. The key to the deep belly breathing technique is to breathe deeply from the belly, getting as much fresh air as possible in your lungs. When you take deep breaths from the abdomen, rather than shallow breaths from your upper chest, you inhale more oxygen. The more oxygen you get, the less tense, short of breath, and anxious you feel.

To begin, sit comfortably with your back straight. Put one hand on your chest and the other on your belly. Slowly take a deep breath in through your nose so that the hand on your belly rises higher than the hand on your chest. The belly should expand, and the hand on the chest should rise very little. Then exhale through your mouth and push out all the air you can while pulling in your belly. Continue to breathe deeply in through your nose and out through your mouth. Try to inhale enough so that your belly rises and falls. Between 1 and 5 minutes of this technique are enough to experience benefits, but feel free to practice as long as you like.

Progressive muscle relaxation

Progressive muscle relaxation is a technique in which you systematically tense and relax different muscle groups. I often teach this exercise at the end of my group fitness classes when the participants are cooling down post workout.

To begin, find a comfortable position sitting or lying down. When you're relaxed and ready to start, shift your attention to your right foot. Take a moment to focus on the way it feels. Slowly tense the muscles in your right foot, squeezing as tightly as you can. Hold for a count of 10. Relax your right foot. Focus on the tension flowing away and the way your foot feels as it becomes limp and loose. Stay in this relaxed state for a moment, breathing deeply and slowly. When you're ready, shift your attention to your left foot. Follow the same sequence of muscle tension and release. Move slowly up through your body, contracting and relaxing all the different muscle groups as you go. I like to begin with the feet and work up to the face, but you can go in whatever order works for you. This technique can take as little as 5 minutes or as long as you like.

Alternate nostril breathing

I learned this breathing technique from my favorite yoga instructor, Stephanie Snyder. *Nadi shodhana*, or alternate nostril breathing, has a long history in Ayurvedic medicine and yoga, where it's thought to harmonize the two hemispheres of the brain, resulting in physical, mental, and emotional balance and well-being.

To begin, sit in any comfortable position. Relax the body and breathe naturally for a few moments, allowing your mind and body to settle. Rest your left hand on your lap or knee. Take your right hand and place the thumb on the right nostril and the index finger or ring finger on the left nostril. Close your eyes. Begin by softly closing your right nostril with your right thumb to inhale slowly, deeply, and smoothly through your left nostril. Then close your left nostril (using your ring or pinky finger) to exhale slowly through your right nostril. Continue in this pattern, inhaling through your right nostril and exhaling through your left. Move through this breathing technique for as long as you wish. When you are finished, relax both arms, sit, and breathe naturally for a few moments before opening your eyes.

Try a few of these techniques, and I think you'll find that the conscious act of breathing is a powerful antidote to stress. When I'm trying to fall asleep after a busy day, get focused for a big presentation, perform well during a workout, or even stay patient during a crowded grocery store trip, I use deep breathing exercises. These simple tools provide powerful results and have enabled me to be my best under stress.

Ease Your Mind

Create mental space.

All the thoughts running around in your head will make you feel overstretched and overstressed. You can't find clarity or focus with all that clutter taking up your head space! Write everything down on paper—I call it a brain dump. From this list of thoughts, you can assess what needs to take priority and then create the mental space to take focused action. This will allow you to feel better able to handle everything. Whatever worries keep your mind busy, write them down on paper and get them out there. It may sound simple, but getting your worry out of your head and into the world will actually help you clear your mind.

Gather a support group.

When you're burned out, you might feel like isolating yourself in order to protect what little energy you have left. But your friends and family are essential in your road to a balanced life. Turn to your loved ones for support. Simply sharing your feelings with another person can relieve stress and ease your anxious mind. The other person doesn't have to fix your problems—he or she just has to be a good listener. Having the right people to connect with will give you lots of moral support, and you'll feel less alone. You can get a fresh perspective and the encouragement you need to take care of yourself.

Watch your thoughts.

In fact, much of what we say to ourselves when experiencing stress can cause us to feel more anxious. Instead, use calming self-talk. Work on practicing empowering, stress-relieving phrases such as "This will pass." "I will get through this." "I am safe." "I am calm." "I am relaxed." Find an affirmation, mantra, or phrase that feels right to you, and repeat it to drown out negative self-talk when feeling stressed. Remember: stress comes from the way you react, not the way life is. The meaning of everything in your life is the meaning you give it. Watch your thoughts and remind yourself that you get to decide what matters and what doesn't.

Just say no.

Don't overextend yourself. Learn how to say no to requests on your time such as happy hour, hosting a fund-raiser, demanding girlfriends, and babysitting a neighbor's pets. Work on saying no to what stresses you out. Give yourself the permission to focus on what's important. Having only essential responsibilities on your schedule will provide you with some extra time and space, and it will lighten the burden you're feeling to keep up with the nonessentials. If you find this difficult, remind yourself that saying no allows you to say yes to what you truly want to do. I go by this rule: "If it's not an absolute yes, then it is a no." Remember: sometimes you have to do what's best for you and your life, not what's best for everyone else.

Practice the STOP Technique.

The STOP technique is a simple strategy to help you pause and get centered. The four letters stand for the following:

S = Stop.
T = Take three deep breaths.
O = Observe the feelings in your body.
P = Move forward and practice gratitude and compassion for yourself and others.

I'm a big advocate of the simple act of taking 3 seconds to check in with your breathing and state of being. By simply taking a moment to do this, you can move forward from a responsive, centered place instead of a reactive one. I also strongly believe that no matter what, acting from a place of gratitude and compassion can help you overcome obstacles.

Download and de-stress.

Here are a few great stress-management resources you can download and use right away.

Meditation and Relaxation Resources

Put your iPhone on airplane mode and take some time to unwind with a guided meditation. I especially love The Mindfulness App, Headspace, and Simply Being for inner peace and calm on the go. Headspace is a personal favorite, the guide's British accent makes me smile and instantly de-stress.

I also like the following apps.

Centered

The Centered app includes everything you need to develop mindfulness skills, including daily reminders, meditation timers, and audio guides of various lengths. You can also sync Centered to Apple Health to help you keep track of your mind, body, and soul in once place. (Free for iOS, itunes.apple.com/us/app/centered)

Zenify

Zenify is a highly useful and varied app that helps you develop mindfulness to cope with stress, be decisive, improve communication skills, be more compassionate and aware of others, and create a more positive inner balance. The app sends you simple assignments to help you practice various skills and incorporate mindfulness into your daily routine. (iOS and Android, zenifyapp.com)

Stop, Breathe, and Think

This well-designed app helps you check in with your state of mind and ease into a meditation routine. The app focuses on developing a strong sense of kindness and compassion by training you to approach yourself and others with a sense of calm. (Free for iOS, for Android, and on the Internet, stopbreathethink.org)

Breathing Zone

Breathing is one of the most important parts of a good stress-management practice. Try beginning your workout with a simple 5-minute breathing exercise using this app, an effective guide to mindful breathing. The soothing visualizer function shows the in-out pattern of the breath with a colorful flowerlike graphic. (itunes.apple.com/us/app/breathing-zone-relaxing-breathing)

Calm

True to its name, Calm is designed to reduce stress and bring a little more calm into users' lives. The app offers a seven-step program designed to give users the tools they need to become calmer, in addition to seven guided relaxation sessions (ranging from 2 to 30 minutes) and ten beautiful and calming nature scenes that users choose to use as wallpapers for their phone. The guided relaxation sessions allow users to bring some Zen into their life at any time of day, and the 2-minute option pretty much eliminates all excuses not to chill out. (calm.com)

Sleep Cycle

Waking up is hard enough, but this app makes it a little less traumatic by analyzing users' sleep patterns and rousing them when they're in the lightest phase of sleep. Plus users get to go through troves of data showing how well (or poorly) they slept during the night. Most sleep-tracking devices are pretty pricey and involve some fancy headgear. But Sleep Cycle's just about the app. Users place their smartphones in bed with them and the app senses what phase of sleep they're in, based on how much or how little they're moving. (sleepcycle.com)

Equanimity

This sleek app was designed in 2009 with the goal of helping the world meditate. To that end, the app provides users with tools to time their sittings, journal post-meditation thoughts and observations, and track their meditation schedules via several useful graphs. Easy-to-use tracking tools allow users to monitor their meditation schedule and quickly notice when they're slipping out of a routine, which makes it that much easier to get back into one. The simple design helps users maintain their Zen post meditation. (meditate.mx/iphone)

iCouch

Here's a tool to help you cope with stressful situations, without having to trek all the way to a therapist's office. The app draws on strategies from the school of cognitive behavioral therapy, an approach that focuses on shifting our thought patterns to be more positive. (icouch.me)

Withings

Withings draws on the basics to monitor wellness. The clear display helps users monitor weekly progress toward long-term goals. Withings also helps keep track of other stats, such as blood pressure and sleep, via other apps like RunKeeper, Bodymedia, and Zeo. (withings.com/us/en)

Here are a some more online resources for relaxation.

You Really Need to Relax: Effective Methods (PDF)
Includes progressive muscle relaxation and relaxation through visual imagery. (University of Michigan Health Center)

Oprah & Deepak Chopra's Meditation Master Trilogy
Three series of 21-day online meditation challenges, which have attracted nearly two million participants.

Chopra Center Meditation Podcast
Resources for aspiring and experienced meditators, including a collection of 24 free meditation podcasts. To bring more mindfulness into your day, you can download the podcasts on iTunes and listen to them at home, on your commute, or while out on a walk.

Movement of Spiritual Awareness online meditation classes
Free online course on meditation and other spiritual resources consisting of readings, audio, and video.

Do Nothing for 2 Minutes
Simple, effective, 2-minute guided visualization break from your day, available for free.

Mindfulness Based Stress Reduction (MBSR)
Dr. Jon Kabat-Zinn developed the Mindfulness Based Stress Reduction (MBSR) program at the University of Massachusetts Medical Center. Since its inception, MBSR has evolved into a common form of complementary medicine addressing a variety of health problems. MBSR is an intensive training in mindfulness meditation, based on ancient healing practices, which meets once a week for 8 weeks. The program brings meditation

and yoga together so that the virtues of both can be experienced simultaneously.

Stress Management Resources (Mind Tools)
This site is divided into 12 sections, laid out nicely and clearly on the main page of the resource. Sections include Understanding Stress, Your Environment, Building Defenses, Avoid Burnout, and more.

Guided Body Scan Meditation
Free 10-minute body scan meditation that can also be downloaded for use on an MP3 player.

MindBody Lab–Audio Relaxation Tracks
A selection of audio relaxation exercises from the University of Texas Counseling and Mental Health Center. Download the tracks at the bottom of the page or access the individual exercises here:

- Muscle Relaxation Exercise
  18-minute progressive muscle relaxation audio exercise (University of Texas Counseling and Mental Health Center).
- Forest Imagery Visualization Exercise
  19-minute visualization audio exercise that guides you through forest imagery (University of Texas Counseling and Mental Health Center).
- Cruise Imagery Visualization Exercise
  12-minute visualization audio exercise that guides you through the imagery of a relaxing cruise (University of Texas Counseling and Mental Health Center).
- Mindful Meditation Audio Exercises
  Free mindful meditations available to play online or as an mp3 download; depending on your browser, may be

easy or challenging to access (UCLA Mindful Awareness Research Center).

• Download Meditations
Download or stream a dozen free meditation recordings to help you cope with life's inevitable hurdles. Comes with handouts (Sitting Together).

PUTTING IT ALL TOGETHER: BALANCED MIND

To improve your ability to manage stress in your life, personalize the preceding suggestions and put them into action. If you practice these techniques routinely, you'll master the art and science of handling stress and be able to beat burnout before it starts. Every day brings you a choice: to practice stress or to practice peace. This chapter showed you that finding peace and sustaining a strong relationship to self doesn't require hours of daily practice. All it takes is a little willingness and commitment to be good to yourself. Life is a precious gift to be savored, not an endless series of chores to complete while you complain about being "crazy busy."

Remember: your to-do list is immortal. It will live on long after you're dead. You may feel like the stress in your life is out of your control, but you can always control the way you respond. Managing stress is all about taking charge: taking charge of your thoughts, your emotions, your schedule, your environment, and the way you deal with problems. Stress management involves changing the stressful situation when you can, changing your reaction when you can't, taking care of yourself, and making time for rest and relaxation. This is your life, and you can choose peace.

Exercise Awareness

Like any muscle, the mind needs regular exercise to stay positive. The stress of our fast-paced world makes it even more challenging to remain mentally grounded, strong, and grateful. In this chapter you found the tools you can use to get your mind in great shape and attract positive outcomes in your life. Now let's work through a few exercises, put all the concepts you learned in this chapter together, and do some mental push-ups.

Take a few minutes to write the answers to the following questions: What are the thoughts that currently shape your mind-set, actions, and outcomes? List a few thoughts you have on a regular basis. How do they affect your actions? How do they affect the outcomes in your life? Now respond to those answers by answering these questions: What would you like to replace those thoughts with? How would this improve your mental health? How would it improve how you relate to yourself? How would it improve how you relate to others? How would it improve your life overall?

The Positive Thought Diet

When you are tempted to criticize, critique, or compare, STOP yourself. Change your thought and replace it with a positive one. Focus on something you are proud of, like how strong your legs feel running 4 miles or how proud you are of yourself for eating a healthy breakfast. Your mind might resist you at first—and will try to keep feeding you negative thoughts, so practice. Build a strong resistance to negative thinking. Don't tolerate trash talk in your life. Making this mental shift is not a quick and easy fix. It takes constant work and awareness, but it is worth it. When you stop beating yourself up, your body and life will show it. You will glow from the inside out. Believe it or not, you might just be able to find the healthy weight, active lifestyle, balance, and wellness that have been waiting for you.

Positive Affirmations

Use the power of positive affirmations to train a more powerful mind. Write three powerful and affirming statements that empower you to achieve the wellness vision you created for yourself in chapter 1. Write your affirmation somewhere you can see it daily and often. Better yet, use your affirmation as a phone reminder, calendar reminder, or computer backdrop.

Gratitude

From the suggestions on adopting a gratitude practice, which works best for you? Do you want to write down three things you are grateful for before bed, take a daily thank-you Instagram photo, or have a weekly time when you observe the gifts in your life? Find a consistent thank-you habit. I like to think of three things I'm grateful for on my walk to get coffee in the morning. By the time I'm at the coffee shop, I'm smiling and in a wonderfully positive mood. It helps me start my day on the right foot. Gratitude is such a powerful tool! Use it!

Minimize Stress

You are the hero of your own story. Find a few stress-management techniques that work for you and practice them consistently. Make them part of your daily routine and part of your lifestyle change. Be proactive, preventive, and take action. Save yourself from stress, and power up your life.

If you've consistently made efforts to improve your mental and emotional health and you still don't feel good, it might be time for professional help. Seek a therapist, coach, or neutral professional party to help you in your health. Input from a knowledgeable, caring professional can enable you to do things for yourself that you might not feel ready to do on your own. Here are a few signs that it might be a good choice:

• Inability to sleep
• Feeling down, hopeless, or helpless most of the time
• Concentration problems that are interfering with your work or home life
• Using nicotine, food, drugs, or alcohol to cope with difficult emotions
• Negative or self-destructive thoughts or fears that you can't control
• Thoughts of death or suicide

If you identify with any of these red-flag symptoms, consider making an appointment with a mental health professional. Know that it's okay to want help. You deserve to live a life that feels good from the inside out.

You can eat right, exercise, and sleep all you want, but you can't have a healthy life without a healthy mind. What does keeping your mind in shape really mean? It means striving to be positive, present, and grateful. It means taking time for self-care and making mental space to find clarity. It means discovering interior barriers and finding the courage to dissolve them. It means learning to be gentle with yourself, love yourself, approve of yourself, and enjoy your life. Keeping your mind in shape is a daily work in progress that takes commitment, consistency, and effort. But trust me: you are worth every ounce of sweat.

I believe from experience that positive thoughts create positive results and that when your mind is in a good place your life will follow suit. Are you ready to get your mind in shape, beat burnout, and fully experience life? The happiness of your life starts with the quality of your thoughts. Use the suggestions in this chapter to train a strong mind, strengthen positive thoughts, and live in health from the inside out.

PART IV

Balanced Spirit

Do you ever feel like the days and weeks just pass you by? Or are you longing to find a deeper sense of belonging with others and the world you live in? Maybe you feel frustrated, disconnected, or scatterbrained. You want a way to find a real sense of meaning so that you can feel driven, motivated, and like you're on a clear path and living the life you want.

It sounds like your spirit may be a little out of shape. Sometimes the best way to heal your life is not figuring out how to work harder but taking time to slow down and enjoy life more. Picture yourself at your ninetieth birthday party with all of your friends and family in attendance. Each person stands up to make a toast to you. What do you want them to say about you? "Joe is a great guy because he owned a Lamborghini" or "Joe has always been able to maintain strong, loving relationships in his life"? "Karen is wonderful because she always stayed thin" or "Karen has led a life filled with curiosity, adventure, and enthusiasm"?

When you find yourself overworked you have to step back, press pause, and get quiet. Sit with yourself and gain some perspective on your life. Why are you working so hard? What matters most to you? How do you want to live your life? What do you want to remember? It's time to improve your spiritual fitness and coach your soul back to health!

Keeping your spirit in shape means pursuing the journey of intentional self-growth. Spiritual fitness is the constant evolution of creating a better version of yourself so that you can make a difference in your life and the lives around you. In fact, the word *spirituality* comes from the Latin root *spiritis*, meaning "breath" and referring to the breath of life. Spirituality deals with the transcendent, intangible dimension of existence that gives us life. Most people value or desire a spiritual element in their lives, but perhaps not in a traditional religious format. Spiritual fitness in this book means maintaining the health of your soul so that you can live with clarity and purpose. Don't worry if your spiritual fitness isn't something you can easily sum up or define. You are spiritual if you are invested in doing the daily work to live consciously and experience your life from a deeper place.

Know that developing spiritual fitness isn't an easy or straightforward process. It's often hard, scary, challenging, vulnerable, and dark. But that is part of the journey. It will often be tough. You will find strength through choosing to persevere and stay the course. Your commitment to your spiritual fitness will allow you to gain control of life's ups and downs. It will allow you to live purely in the mind-set of growth and change. It will fuel your ability to grow better even when life becomes challenging, and it will empower you to leave burnout behind.

Remember: happiness is not a destination but a manner of traveling. Your course is not defined. It's not a path on a map that you follow. Instead it's waking up daily with the intention to be better than the day before. You are a constantly evolving work in progress, and keeping your spirit in shape will help keep you on course in living a meaningful life.

When you nurture the health of your spirit, you can steer your life forward toward positive results. You can feel centered, grounded, intentional, powerful, and focused. This takes consistent commitment and work, but it is possible—and you can start now.

What do you do to take care of yourself and to keep yourself centered? What do you do to find meaning and stay connected to the world you live in? In chapters 9, 10, and 11, I'll be giving you my top exercises for a healthier spirit. There are so many different ways to nurture your spiritual health. This is not a comprehensive list, just a few suggestions to help you to connect to yourself in a way that fills you up and gives you the strength to climb out of burnout. Through a regular reflection practice, strengthening your self-esteem, maintaining meaningful social relationships, dedicating time to play, giving back, and present-moment living, I believe you will develop a spiritual workout plan that will enable you to live with intention, purpose, and fulfillment. Get ready to rediscover what makes you feel alive.

CHAPTER 9

Reflection: Go Inward and Go Often

It is only when we silence the blaring sounds of our daily existence that we can finally hear the whispers of truth that life reveals to us, as it stands knocking on the doorsteps of our hearts.
—K. T. Jong

My whole life I've loved the art of reflection. I have journals from when I was in elementary school, documenting details of my days, dreams, and goals. In fact, it was my daily practice of reflection that empowered me to leave my negative habits and burnout behind. Day after day, I saw my unhappiness stare back at me from the pages of my journal entries. Each note of stress brought me more awareness to the fact that how I was living wasn't working for me. The longer I sat with that fact and my feelings, the more I knew it was time for a change. Then came the journal entry where I knew it was time. I was ready to take action and take back my life.

You must find a way to connect with yourself on a daily and consistent basis in order to live an intentional life. You don't have to write in a journal—you just need to find a habit that works for you. Read, write, go for a hike, sit outside and meditate—but develop a ritual that allows you to regularly go inward.

A reflection practice offers you an opportunity to get away from the voices of others and connect to your own. It gives you a break from the have-to's and allows you to focus on the want-to's. It lets you address your own needs and helps you pause to check in with your life.

We have grown to appreciate the art of getting to know others, but it is even more important to get to know ourselves, our preferences, and our likes and dislikes, without other people's influence. Reflection allows you the opportunity to discover things about yourself and to get a real understanding of who you are. A reflection practice will help you clear your mind and weed through your thoughts. It will allow you to get to the heart of what you really think as opposed to being told or influenced by others and their opinions. It gives you time to reflect on what is important in your life and how you feel about situations that need to be addressed.

By spending time with yourself and gaining a better understanding of who you are and what you desire in life, you're more likely to make better choices about who and what you want to be around. I know it can be a challenge to find time alone in a world that seems to never sleep. But you deserve some attention and a strong relationship to your inner self.

DEVELOPING A REFLECTION PRACTICE

Here are a few great ways to personalize a reflection practice and spend quality one-on-one time with yourself:

Exercise solo.
Go for a walk, run, swim, or bike ride. You can even leave the headphones at home and spend time listening to your thoughts and the world.

Journal.
I spend a lot of time journaling and love to use my journal time for reflection, goal setting, and creating positive intentions for my life.

Meditate.
It doesn't have to be for long. Sit still with yourself. Watch your thoughts—no judgment. Review the meditation guides and resources in chapter 8.

Take yourself on a date.
Try dinner, a movie, or a museum. Embrace being out with yourself alone.

Have a self-care night.
Block out the time in your schedule, then unplug from all tech, work, and people. Take a bath, read, pamper yourself. Do whatever you like!

Get lost.
Go for a walk, hike, or drive somewhere you've never been before. Explore.

Get crafty or creative.
Paint, create, take photos, make a vision board. There are so many ways to get creative and express yourself while spending time alone.

Get up and get it in early.
This is probably the ideal way to find and spend some time alone to reflect. When you wake up before the rest of the world, you can carve out peaceful, uninterrupted downtime. Instead of waking up late and rushing to work, you'll start your day grounded and calm. The peace of the early morning reflection practice is addicting. Some of the activities that you can do to enjoy spending time alone in the morning include writing, learning something new, reading, watching an inspiring video, meditating, exercising, walking, having coffee, thinking and reflecting, or listening to music.

PUTTING IT ALL TOGETHER: THE INNER JOURNEY

It's important to remember that the reflection practices you choose to do should allow you to be real, open, and vulnerable. Keeping your spirit in shape means allowing yourself to feel, to experience deeply all the ups and downs of life. This means you've got to find a way to let yourself express and release your true feelings. A powerful reflection practice is a channel for you to be open and honest with yourself. It gives you space to acknowledge and work on yourself in a loving, self-helping way. This will allow you to strengthen your spirit and continue to pursue the path of personal growth.

We live in a demanding world, and we demand much of ourselves. The harder we push, the more time we need to reconnect to ourselves. Take action now: stop and find a way to connect to your inner self consistently in your life. Slow down. Breathe. Give yourself permission to pause, regroup, and move forward with clarity and purpose.

CHAPTER 10
Self-Esteem and Self-Care

The moment you doubt whether you can fly, you cease forever to be able to do it.
—Peter Pan

Self-esteem is the opinion you hold of yourself—your self-acceptance rating. No matter how many other people think you are fabulous, if you don't believe in yourself, that will negatively impact your health. When you have low-self esteem, you are more likely to do the following:

- Work more than is good for you despite being exhausted or in bad health
- Ignore your own needs and wishes and devote your time to other activities and people
- Tolerate a situation that is directly hurting you on a personal level and take no action to improve it

Strengthening your self-esteem and loving yourself will allow you to leave the cycle of burnout. So what can you do to turn low-esteem behaviors around to start acting and feeling more like yourself again? Plenty. The good news is that self-esteem is a skill that can be learned and nurtured. Like any other skill, it involves understanding specific actionable steps and practicing them until you get stronger. Let's start the self-esteem exercise now!

STRENGTHENING YOUR SELF-ESTEEM

Here are some ways to strengthen your self-esteem:

Take risks.
Are you a risk taker? Are you the kind of person who doesn't fear failure? The more willing you are to put yourself out there, take risks, and overcome fears, the more you will strengthen your self-esteem. List a few risks that you want to take. Maybe they are related to the wellness vision you created in chapter 1. What are the fears that are holding you back? What will you gain if you take this risk? What will you lose if you take this risk? Take a deep breath and go for it! Don't be afraid to feel uncomfortable. Don't be afraid to look uneasy and a little silly in front of others. It's all about your commitment to learning, adapting, and growing. Decide that your visions and goals are more important than your fears. Dare to try. Step outside of your comfort zone. Believe you can, and you're halfway there.

Exercise your confidence.
If you feed your confidence, you'll starve your fears. Have you ever heard the expression "Fake it until you make it"? In small and manageable situations, practice acting confidently, even if

you don't feel confident yet. Speak up in a meeting. Introduce yourself to someone new. Challenge yourself to do something a bit beyond your comfort zone. As you take action and see some success in these smaller situations, you'll feel more and more confident. Your increased confidence will allow you to tackle riskier actions that have a higher payoff in the long run.

Avoid comparison.

Comparison is the thief of joy. It is a deadly trap that we all often fall into. If you want to strengthen your healthy self-esteem, stop comparing yourself. The only life you get to live is your own. The sooner you accept that and drop the comparison trap, the happier you'll be. When you question yourself, your value, or your worth, you are undermining every gift you were given. It's like you are saying "You didn't make me good enough, so I have to look out there for proof." If you believe you aren't good enough, you'll find ways to prove to yourself that you aren't. If you believe you are good enough, you'll find ways to prove to yourself that you are. Stop comparing and start believing in yourself now.

Stop putting yourself down.

How do you talk to yourself? What do you focus on? Get in the habit of focusing on your positive qualities. Stop beating yourself up! The way you treat yourself sets the standard for others. You must love who you are or no one will.

Accept compliments and celebrate your successes.

Being proud isn't bragging about how great you are. Being proud is quietly knowing that you're worth a lot. It's not about thinking you're perfect but about knowing that you're worthy of being loved and accepted. You can boost your self-esteem by recognizing your accomplishments and celebrating them.

Acknowledge your positive qualities, and when you come across a quality in yourself that you aren't proud of, work pro-actively on correcting it.

Approach challenges.
Overcoming challenges and obstacles will strengthen your resilience and self-esteem. Remember: it's all about attitude. Look at every obstacle as a chance to grow into a stronger version of you.

Associate with confident and successful people.
Ever notice how negative, unhappy people suck the life right out of you? Surround yourself with people who lift you higher. When you are around smart, accomplished, supportive, happy people, you'll feel better about yourself and will become a happy person for it. Be around those who bring out the best in you, not the stress in you.

Set aside a time each day for personal development.
A stronger spirit comes from your commitment to personal growth. How much you grow and who you become is up to you. Remember: the acquisition of knowledge doesn't mean you're growing; growing happens when what you know changes how you live.

The reality is that we are all uniquely fabulous and abundantly talented. It's up to us to decide how much to cultivate and how much to shine. Confidence is believing in yourself. You can choose right here and now to believe. We have all had failures and challenges. But those who keep believing in themselves despite theses experiences are the ones who succeed in the long run.

Make today—and every day—a brand new start. Learn from your failures, and grow better because of them. Each time you choose to take action toward a stronger version of yourself, your confidence and self-esteem will grow. Keep telling yourself how special you are. Strengthen your belief in you!

SHIFT YOUR SELF-CARE PERCEPTION FOR A HEALTHIER SPIRIT

When I loved myself enough, I began leaving whatever wasn't healthy. This meant people, jobs, my own beliefs, and habits—anything that kept me small. My judgment called it disloyal. Now I see it as self-loving.
—*Kim McMillen*

Self-care seems like a simple concept, yet it really isn't, is it? It's a challenge for us all. Before hitting burnout, I was the worst at self-care. For years I helped my clients achieve their goals and put myself on the bottom of my priorities. By 2011 I was exhausted, injured, and resentful. It may seem admirable to work yourself sick, but the longer you burn the candle at both ends and put yourself last, the faster you'll reach a breaking point. That's what happened to me. I broke. Then I woke up.

At first, making myself a priority to leave burnout was incredibly scary. It took courage to be self-compassionate and to acknowledge that I needed support in being the best version of myself. I learned that I needed to accept my own imperfections, face my challenges, and love myself enough to be the number-one priority in my life. To do this, you have to get rid of any limiting beliefs that may be holding you back. The following are some of the myths about self-care that can prevent you from giving yourself the love you need to reach your full potential.

MYTHS AND REALITIES OF SELF-CARE

Myth 1: Self-care is selfish.
Many of us are taught to care for everyone except ourselves. Self-care can be seen as selfish—that taking care of yourself means you are not doing what you are supposed to be doing, which is taking care of someone else.

Reality: Caring for others requires loving kindness and authenticity. If you haven't created those traits for yourself, how can you give them to others? I found that through caring for myself I was a better coach, friend, daughter, sister, and person. It may seem counterintuitive at first, but you truly can give more to others when you take care of yourself first.

> *Self-care is never a selfish act—it is simply good stewardship of the only gift I have, the gift I was put on earth to offer to others.*
> *—Parker Palmer*

Myth 2: Self-care is indulgent.
You might be concerned that being nice to yourself lets you off the hook and encourages you to be self-indulgent.

Reality: Self-care is about your health and well-being, whereas self-indulgence is about getting anything you want when you want it without thoughts of well-being. Self-care is about noticing and dealing with your pain. Self-indulgence is about numbing and denying your pain.

Self-care is not about self-indulgence. It's about self-preservation.
—Audre Lorde

Myth 3: Self-criticism is what motivates you.

Self-love is often devalued. Instead we often use self-criticism to motivate us to reach our goals. Self-criticism can work to motivate us to a certain extent, but it creates a lot of trouble in doing so: guilt, shame, fear of failure, thoughts of not being good enough, and fear of humiliation, just to name a few. Self-criticism also provides the illusion of control. If you just worked harder, looked prettier, or acted nicer, you could achieve that perfection you've been seeking, right? You know the answer to that question, but the pursuit of perfection and the lure of control are hard to shake in our attempts to care for ourselves.

Reality: While it's possible the inner critic developed to help you reach your goals, it's not the only option. We have many ways to keep ourselves moving forward. We really don't need a critical voice in our heads to do so. We don't need to be internally nagged and disparaged to accomplish things. Being self-compassionate gives you the confidence you need to motivate yourself in a positive way.

You have been criticizing yourself for years, and it hasn't worked. Try approving of yourself and see what happens.
—Louise L. Hay

Myth 4: Self-compassion is wimpy.

In our individualistic society, you are supposed to "pull yourself up by your bootstraps" and tough things out. Be kind to yourself? Quit being such a wimp!

Reality: Actually, self-compassion serves to heal and strengthen you. It is, in fact, the strongest and most resilient among us who have the courage to be kind to ourselves.

These are just a few of the limiting beliefs that can prevent you from practicing self-care and beating burnout. Can you pinpoint any ideas you have about taking care of yourself that keep you in a cycle of putting yourself last?

PUTTING IT ALL TOGETHER: SELF-CARE FOR A STRONGER SPIRIT

Maybe you have been taught to ignore, deny, or suppress your personal wants or needs due to believing any or all the preceding myths, but now you are ready to beat burnout and change your mind-set to support yourself in doing it! Practice noticing your personal desires, and gently give yourself validation that they are real and deserve compassion. Do you have the desire to spend more time with friends? Do you want to work with someone on improving your fitness or nutrition? Do you want to take up a hobby or spend more time relaxing? What is it that you want for your life (not the life of your friend, client, or daughter)? Is there something that you always wish you had the time to do? Make it happen now. And make it happen for yourself.

As you work to leave burnout behind, treat yourself as you would a friend. Speak gently to yourself. Be understanding. Don't tolerate negative or critical self-talk. Talk to yourself as you would someone you love. Even if you are going through a challenge or make mistakes, be gentle, forgiving, and kind to yourself. You're human! All of us are flawed, make mistakes, and are deserving of love. Perfection doesn't exist. Let go and learn to love your beautifully imperfect self.

> *And now that you don't have to be perfect, you can be good.*
> —*John Steinbeck*

When you start to believe that you are worth taking time for, then you will take action toward giving yourself the time and attention you need to live well. It's time to make yourself a priority and find the balanced life you deserve.

CHAPTER 11

Connect to Yourself and Your World

Living a fulfilling and meaningful life requires you to figure out what is fulfilling and meaningful to you. Take the time and energy to discover what you're passionate about and what gives you a sense of purpose. This might take some time and research, but it is well worth it. Once you figure it out, spend as much time as possible doing those things. If you can make it your career or part of your career, that's all the better.

Don't be too hard on yourself if you haven't defined your passions yet. No one is judging you or pressuring you to claim a set list of things you love. You have a lifetime for exploring new joys. Don't worry about picking one—just give yourself permission to discover what makes you happy and be a lifetime learner of whatever makes your heart smile.

Spend some time thinking about what you love to do. What areas of life are you naturally drawn to? What do you love to do when you have free time? What gives you a real buzz of excitement? If you had five years left to live, what would you do? If you inherited $300 million, how would it change your life? What would you choose to do with your days? What interests you that you would love to know more about? Give yourself time to uncover what makes you feel alive, and find ways to make those passions a regular part of your life.

PLAY

One of my friends is an expert at play. He dedicates time in his life to leisure, fun, adventure, and new experiences. He works hard at accomplishing his goals and has a very successful career, but he also respects and values the art of play. His enthusiasm is contagious. He brings energy and zest with him everywhere he goes. I find myself continuously inspired by his love of life. His example reminds me that success isn't determined by accolades or accomplishments. Rather, success is determined by how happy you are and how much fun you are having.

The element of play was nonexistent in my life when I was burned out. I didn't make time for any fun. I was too focused on getting ahead. If I did anything remotely like play, it was scheduled and strict. There wasn't really any letting go and enjoying of the moment. At the time, I thought this made me driven and dedicated, but really it was self-sabotage. All work and no play is the fast track to burnout. Post wake-up call, I'm learning to let go. I make time for and enjoy leisure!

Play is not a luxury. It is a necessity in living a balanced life. Playing gives you the balance you need to deal with non leisure activities such as work, bills, cleaning, and errands. It provides you with needed relief from stress, thereby promoting better physical and mental health. *Not* playing makes you an illness-prone, stressed, burned-out mess.

You cannot call your life balanced if all you do is work. Maybe you don't think play is that important, or you think you already use your leisure time well. Maybe you feel guilty taking time off to play or have been working so much you've forgotten *how* to play. It's time to give yourself permission to relax, play, and do goofy stuff. Your health depends on it. Here are a few ways to bring play back into your life.

Take a play day.
Give yourself a play day—a whole day away from work and responsibilities, dedicated to the sole purpose of having fun. It would be ideal if you left your phone at home or put it on airplane mode. It's always a good idea to ask others to join you on your day of play. Go for a hike, have a long lunch somewhere nice, or sit by a pool and read a good book—whatever you like. It should feel like a mini vacation. You might like it so much you'll start a play-day tradition.

Say yes to something new.
Choose an activity you've never done before, something out of your comfort zone. It doesn't need to be something as edgy as skydiving. It can be as simple as learning to cook a new dish or attending a local concert. Expanding your repertoire of favorite activities keeps play fresh and fun. There are so many things to try. Get out there and give yourself a new experience that gives you joy.

Make a list of things you want to do.
Then do them! You can make a goal to cross one off the list each day, week, month, or year.

Be assured that surfing on Instagram or winning Candy Crush Saga does not count as real leisure time. Put down your smartphone and go play! Check out the facilities and schedules of your local recreation department, theater, meetups, and more.

If you love hiking and the last time you went was four years ago. . . .If you love cooking and the last time you made a meal was 2012. . . . If swimming makes you happy, but you haven't been in the water since your second kid was born. . . . I challenge you to change that. Prevent early aging and give yourself permission to put play back into your life.

"We don't stop playing because we grow old; we grow old because we stop playing."
—*George Bernard Shaw*

MEANINGFUL SOCIAL RELATIONSHIPS

Do you never have time for your friends, then feel empty when there's no one to hang out with? Or do you wish you had someone to be real with, someone who "gets it"? When you are struggling with burnout, making time for your relationships may feel like the last thing you have energy for, but maintaining meaningful personal relationships can support you back to balance and keep your spirit in good shape. After all, it's not always where you are in life but who you have by your side that matters. What's the point of being successful without others to share it with? I want you to make the time to nurture and develop quality relationships so that you can experience more happiness, purpose, and health. Real friends and family will bring out the best in you and help with balance too. Longing to find connection and relationships that enhance your well-being? Here are my action steps to grow and maintain meaningful positive relationships in your life.

Take inventory of the relationships you already have.

We accumulate a lot of relationships in our lives. Some of them are meant to last a lifetime, and others are meant to teach us lessons. Not everyone in your life is meant to stay; some are meant to be part of your history, not your destiny. Think through the relationships you have at the moment and notice any that are no longer serving your best interest. To be able to stay positive and healthy it is essential to have influences in your life that support you and lift you up instead of drag you down. You have control. Consciously decide who and what you choose to spend time with. If in doubt, ask yourself "After I leave their company, do I feel energized or drained?" I know that it can be hard to let go when it comes to relationships. We cling to people because they are part of our past, even when we know they are not ideal for us in the present. If you find that some relationships are no longer healthy for you and are draining your energy, it's time to let them go. Remember: letting go of toxic relationships doesn't mean you don't care about these people anymore; it's just that you realize you control who surrounds you and are deciding to choose well. The bottom line is that when you start compromising your happiness and potential for the people around you, you need to change the people around you. Channel your energy toward finding and maintaining healthy, fulfilling relationships. Be with those who bring out the best in you, not the stress in you.

Make the effort.

Relationships don't develop automatically and don't deepen on their own; they take effort. If you want good friends in your life, you must be a good friend. Be aware of this in your relationships, and think about what efforts you can make to deepen your connection with people who matter to you. What kind of effort would be most significant to each individual?

Some people don't care about birthdays, or actually hate being reminded of them, and others feel slighted if they don't get a phone call or an e-card. Pay close attention to what other people value, and make the effort to connect with them on that level.

Every little bit counts.
Think you need a couple hours or a special event to make time spent with a friend worth it? Think again. Every little bit counts when it comes to developing and maintaining relationships. Maybe you choose to multitask with other to-dos on your healthy living life list: share a workout, cook a healthy meal together, share the commute to work, run errands jointly, and so on. You don't need a special occasion to meet up with a friend. Enhance your day-to-day tasks by sharing that time with your friends.

When you have a quality friend, tell them that's how you feel.
Show appreciation for those in your life who bring you joy, community, and friendship.

Spend real time together.
Keeping in touch with people these days through social media comments, e-mails, or text messages is not the same as doing it in real time. Don't let the fact that you've had regular e-contact with someone online replace face-to-face or voice-to-voice time. A little bit of real time is more powerful than anything the Internet can give you. So put down the smartphone, close the laptop, and enjoy each other's company, face-to-face, the old-fashioned way. Few life pleasures equal a good conversation, a genuine laugh, a walk, or a big hug shared by two people who care about each other. Sometimes the most ordinary things can be made extraordinary simply by doing them with

the right people. You know this! Choose to be around these people, and choose to make the most of your time together. Your spirit will soar.

Be honest.
Relationships built on falsehoods or façades are only as stable as their foundation. Superficial relationships will fizzle over time. Seek to create real relationships built on honesty, trust, authenticity, and integrity. Real friends are the ones who know you as you are, understand where you have been, accept who you have become, and still encourage you to grow. To achieve positive relationships that will nourish your spirit seek out those with whom you can be yourself.

Alter your expectations, and don't make assumptions.
In any relationship, we can start to impose on our friends certain expectations that set us up to feel hurt or disappointed. Keep realistic expectations of your friends. Notice when you're projecting something onto the other person that has nothing to do with them, like a fear from a past relationship, and then make an effort to let it go. Recognize when you're looking for that person to do something for you that you need to do for yourself, like making you feel lovable or taking care of your needs, and then release those expectations and do it for yourself. Share the love.

> *At the end of the day people won't remember what you said or did; they will remember how you made them feel.*
> —*Maya Angelou*

It's so true: people don't remember what you say; they remember how you made them feel. Make them feel good.

Supporting, guiding, and making contributions to other people is one of life's greatest rewards. In order to get, you have to give.

Treat everyone with kindness and respect.
People will notice your kindness, and it will most likely produce positive results.

Accept people as they are.
In most cases it's impossible to change people, and it's rude to try. Save yourself from needless stress. Instead of trying to change others, give them your support, love, and acceptance.

Encourage others and cheer for them.
Having an appreciation for how amazing the people around you are leads to productive, fulfilling, and peaceful relationships. Be happy for those who are making progress, and cheer for their victories. Show gratitude, and be openly thankful for others. What goes around comes around, and sooner or later the people you're cheering for will start cheering for you.

Forgive others and let go.
Holding on to resentment is like drinking poison and expecting someone else to die when in fact you end up hurting yourself more than the people you resent. Don't live with hate or anger in your heart. Learn to forgive and let go. Forgiveness is not saying "What you did to me is okay." It is saying "I'm not going to let what you did to me ruin my happiness forever." You're not erasing the past or forgetting what happened. Rather, you're letting go of the resentment and pain and choosing to learn from the incident and move on with your life. Remember: the less time you spend hating the people who hurt you, the more time you'll have to love the people who love you.

Give what you want to receive.

Don't expect what you are not willing to give. Start practicing the Golden Rule. If you want love, give love. If you want good friends, be a good friend. If you want money, provide value. It works. It really is this simple.

Keep your promises, and tell the truth.

It's hard to maintain a relationship with a flake. If you say you're going to do something, honor your commitment. Always be open and honest. Real friends keep promises and tell the truth upfront.

Be your imperfectly perfect self.

In this world that's trying to make you like everyone else, find the courage to keep being your awesome self. People enjoy spending time with others who are happy, content, and confident. Be who you are—and own it. Don't change so people will like you. Be yourself and the right people will love the real you. You'll empower others to do the same.

Work on being the type of person you want to be around.

You must always focus energy inward first. Before befriending others, you have to be your own friend. Before making others happy, you have to make yourself happy. It's not selfishness; it's personal development. And that is what this whole book is about!

Do your relationships have the following characteristics?

- The ability to love and be loved
- Mutual understanding
- Caring
- Honesty
- Trust

- Accountability
- Support
- Encouragement
- Validation of self-worth
- Security
- A diversity of positive ideas and influences to help you grow and learn
- Fun

Take action: Evaluate your relationships. Do they maintain some of the characteristics listed above? Who are the top five people in your life who positively affect your personal growth? What's one habit you can implement to nurture and develop meaningful personal relationships?

Realize that it is less important to have more friends than it is to have real ones. Life is like a party: you invite a lot of people, some leave early, some stay all night, some laugh with you, some laugh at you, and some show up really late, but in the end, after the fun, a few stay to help you clean up the mess. Most of the time, those people aren't even the ones who made the mess. They're your real friends. They're the ones who matter most.

GIVE BACK

There is far too much complaining in this world. We whine when it rains, are upset when the coffee machine is broken, feel annoyed when gas prices go up again. But when we take a moment to remember that there are people who don't have homes to protect them from the weather, who can't afford coffee and can't own a car, our perspective shifts. Suddenly a snag on our new pair of Lululemon capris doesn't seem like such a tragedy.

It's time to stop all the complaining and start contributing to the world in a positive way. I believe doing so fuels spiritual health, happiness, and purpose. Be the change! Let's take collective action and make this world a better place.

Charity played a powerful role in helping me stay grateful, make a positive difference in my world, and recover from burnout. I began by joining local groups and started helping host events to raise awareness and funds for causes I believed in. I met incredible people, made meaningful memories, and got to contribute to something bigger than myself. Today I am still involved in philanthropy and feel incredibly lucky to have the opportunity to give back. I gain perspective on my own life whenever I volunteer. Charity work transforms my attitude and fills my heart. And it's so easy to help. You don't have to take a year off work to make a difference. Find a cause that is near and dear to your heart. Raise awareness, help with funding, attend an event, forward an e-mail. If an issue touches you, do something to help move it forward. When you put good out there, it comes back to you. Here are a few balanced body benefits of giving back:

- Improves mood and self-esteem. Face-to-face helping gives us a "helper's high."
- Reduces excessive self-centeredness (It is not all about you all the time!)
- Reduces social isolation (You meet new and like-minded people.)
- Helps with depression and anxiety
- Improves your social support network while increasing the level of community wellness

- Helps you develop confidence in your own abilities (Yes, you can make a difference!)
- Teaches a variety of new skills

Want to lend a hand but don't know where to begin? Here are a few resources that can help you start.

Instead App

"You don't have to be a billionaire to change the world. You can do it $3 and $5 at a time," the Instead website reads. This "micro donations, macro impact" app is all about tapping into our everyday choices. The app clearly displays the impact of your choice—so in lieu of your regular store-bought coffee, those few dollars could provide a South Sudanese child with clean water for a year. The causes are supported by an Instead nonprofit partner, and the app keeps 5 percent of the donation for operating costs. Donations are tax deductible. (instead.com)

Charity Miles App

Donate without dipping into your bank account and become a sponsored athlete? That's a beautiful thing. Charity Miles is the easiest way to integrate philanthropy into your daily workout by earning money and raising awareness for charities each time you exercise. Just turn on the app, choose a charity, and press start. The app measures the distance of your route. Bikers earn 10 cents per mile, and walkers and runners earn 25 cents per mile, all depending on the Charity Miles corporate sponsorship pool. (charitymiles.org)

One Today App

Google's One Today app lets you "give a little and change a lot" by combining philanthropy with the excitement of novelty. Every day, discover a new nonprofit organization. If you like its mission, you can donate $1 from within the app. For example, you can help adopt a coral reef, save a child from pneumonia, or fund a critical surgical procedure. Through One Today you can share new organizations with friends, or match your friends' donations, which are tax deductible and grouped together for simple year-end tax planning. (onetoday.google.com)

Idealist

This website helps you find a job, internship, or volunteer opportunity based on where you live, your schedule, and your interests. The site helps you get involved in your own community, updating you on ongoing volunteer opportunities, one-time asks from nonprofits, and events in your area. (idealist.org)

All for Good

The largest database of volunteer opportunities online, All for Good is a great platform for finding ways to make a difference. Each month, the site hosts 150,000 local volunteer listings. All for Good is part of Points of Light, the largest volunteer network in the world. (allforgood.org)

DoSomething

More than two million young people have found a cause and started their own volunteer projects through DoSomething, one of the most popular giving platforms. The organization's motto is "We make the world suck less." DoSomething connects you with the resources you need to launch joint initiatives like collecting jeans for homeless youth or donating cell phones to domestic-abuse survivors. (mobileapp.dosomething.org)

Help from Home

This site is committed to helping you "change the world in just your pajamas." Offering ways to micro-volunteer, it connects you with ways to give back at a moment's notice in ways that fit into your schedule. Donate unused air miles with a few clicks, proofread a page of text, or give to a family in need. (helpfromhome.org)

VolunteerMatch

With around 77,000 opportunities to give back, VolunteerMatch connects you to causes and lets you tailor your searches according to what you care about most. You can type in what matters to you in the "I Care About" box. In addition to listing opportunities, the site offers tools that help organizations from corporations to colleges encourage employees and students to volunteer and invite others to participate. (volunteermatch.org)

Do you want to feed a strong spirit? Look for daily opportunities to serve those around you and make the world a better place. We have so many opportunities every day to help others in a simple or grand way. Each time you do so, your own energy increases, you feel great, and you make the world better, bit by bit. Your daily acts of service eventually cascade into a more heartfelt and meaningful life—both for you and those around you.

LIVE IN THE MOMENT: CONSCIOUS LIVING

Breathe deeply and appreciate the moment. Living in the moment could be the meaning of life.
—from the Lululemon manifesto

Think the previous quotation is a bunch of Lululemon fluff? Think again. Believe it or not, the simple act of being in the moment can nourish your spirit and take your health to the next level. In our busy lives we tend to over-plan and under-appreciate. We rarely stop to just be in the moment and enjoy the world around us, whether it be an amazing cup of coffee or the company we keep. It is these little things that truly bring us joy and happiness.

This concept used to be verbalized as "Stop and smell the roses." In today's world, it's more like "Put the phone down and enjoy life." Too often we have our head buried in our smartphones, unaware of life all around us. While it sounds like a great idea to have a video of the event you are attending, wouldn't it be better to actually be in the moment and watch it with your own eyes instead of through your phone? When we learn to live in the moment and experience the world, we realize we are truly blessed. Learning to practice present-moment living will improve your spiritual fitness and allow you to experience joy in your life.

Remember then: there is only one time that is important—now! It is the most important time because it is the only time when we have any power.
—Leo Tolstoy

There are two ways to live life: consciously or unconsciously. Conscious living, or mindful living, implies being an active participant in your life, choosing the experiences you get involved with, and taking responsibility for the decisions you make. The opposite, unconscious living, means allowing circumstances to dictate your life, remaining passive, and taking little to no ownership over what life brings.

When you live consciously, you become intentional in what you do. You put yourself in the driver's seat and, instead of waiting for things to happen, you make things happen. You get more done, are more intentional, and are more focused. All of this gives you the ability to accomplish what you set out to do and allows you to be more successful in life. The best part is that holding yourself accountable for the life you have has a direct and positive impact on self-esteem, attitude, and belief in yourself.

Studies have shown that conscious living provides numerous health benefits. It helps reduce and manage stress, chronic pain, and blood pressure, and it increases immune function and the ability to cope with disease. Individuals who live consciously tend to be happier, take themselves less seriously, be less impulsive or reactive, and accept their own weaknesses without self-judgment, all while having a more positive outlook than those who don't do these things. Further, they're able to take criticism more easily, and they suffer less from depression and other emotional and behavioral issues.

Living consciously also means focusing on the present and not dwelling on the past or obsessing about the future—in other words, living life in the moment. This translates to experiencing more positive thoughts and feelings as most of our anxiety and fears are rooted in past disappointments or regrets and the worry we feel about the future.

Want to savor the journey, not just the destination? Are you ready to be an active participant in your life and live in the moment every day? Living consciously can occur at any moment, on any day, just by actively being present during your experiences and aware of your feelings and emotions. All it takes to get started is a commitment and choice to be present in your life. Here are my guidelines for living in the moment (and actually enjoying it!) so you can strengthen your spirit.

Stop and smell the roses (or put down the phone and enjoy life).

Throughout the day, take time to pay attention to what is happening around you. Become mindful of your environment and how you personally fit into it. Observe colors, sounds, light, smells, and textures. Savor moments by allowing all of your senses to fully experience them. Make a habit of noticing new things in every situation and during daily actions like walking to work and making breakfast. There is so much life to see and savor even in the simplest act.

Experiment and try new things.

Take a class. Attend a seminar. Read a new book. Play a new game. When opportunities present themselves, embrace them openly and look for the potential that they may bring. Say yes instead of no, and do one thing a day that scares you. Trying new things keeps you engaged, youthful, and living to the fullest.

Stop overthinking.

Jon Kabat-Zinn, professor of medicine emeritus and founding executive director of the Stress Reduction Clinic and the Center for Mindfulness in Medicine, Health Care, and Society at the University of Massachusetts Medical School, teaches mindfulness and Mindfulness-Based Stress Reduction (MBSR) in various venues around the world. He tells us, "Ordinary thoughts course through our mind like a deafening waterfall." Part of our inability to live consciously is that we let our thoughts overtake our minds, which prevents us from living in the moment and experiencing life. Instead, allow yourself to "just be." Focus less on your thoughts and more on what's going on around you at the moment. Actively take part in the present while shutting out negativity of the past or future.

Breathe.

When you feel the urge to be impulsive or have a knee-jerk reaction to something, stop and take a few deep, cleansing breaths. When it comes to building a conscious life, deep breathing helps you hit the restart button. Instead of reacting hastily or irrationally, you're able to pause, gain self-control, and have a more intentional response to situations and circumstances. Breathing is free, easy, and doable anywhere, so inhale, exhale, and repeat!

Accept, deal, and overcome challenges, pain, and worry.

When something is uncomfortable, we often feel compelled to avoid it. Instead of pushing negative feelings away, simply allow yourself to feel them and accept them for what they are. When we don't acknowledge negative feelings and try to ignore them, they end up coming back to haunt us. They can manifest in unhealthy behaviors, cause us to do things we may regret, or keep us in a state of unhappiness. When you choose to accept negative feelings, you can gain the understanding and strength to move forward and move past negativity instead of living with it. I always say you have to feel it in order to heal it.

Switch from autopilot to manual.

You know your inner autopilot is at work when you feel like time has passed you by, yet you have no idea what you did or what happened during that time. You are going through the motions instead of actively engaging in your life. Maybe autopilot kicks in during a commute or while running errands. Maybe it occurs at work for longer periods of time. To get the most out of life, be an active participant. Shut off autopilot by increasing your awareness of your thoughts, actions, decisions, and experiences. Don't defer to others to make decisions for you or allow circumstances to dictate your life. Doing so will only lead to disappointment and frustration. Conscious living allows you to choose to be the pilot of your life and to take control of where you go and the direction you head. Look constantly for ways to engage in what life has to offer, and create meaningful moments that you remember.

When you take the time to enjoy the moments of your life, you will experience more joy, happiness, and positive emotions, and fewer of those that are negative or depressing. You don't need me to tell you that conscious living is worthwhile. Being an active participant in your life just feels better!

Take action: Stay grounded in this very moment . . . this breath, this step, this bite, this sound, this person right in front of you. Meaning and fulfillment aren't the result of some complex, hard-won search or found in achieving some large, lofty goal. It's found in who you are being and how you are showing up in each moment. Everything you've been searching for can be found by fully immersing yourself in this moment. If you can do this, you'll find the meaning that has been present all along.

PUTTING IT ALL TOGETHER: BALANCED SPIRIT

Your spirit needs regular exercise if you want a meaningful life. In this chapter I shared some tools you can use to get your spirit in great shape and live with intention and fulfillment. Now let's put it all together and make a spiritual fitness plan that works for you.

Practice reflection.
Find a way to focus inwardly and connect with yourself. Reading this book and working through the exercises can be part of that. Spend regular time alone so that you can step back and continue to create an intentional life.

Boost your self-esteem and embrace self-care.
Exercise your confidence by taking risks, approaching challenges, avoiding comparison, and celebrating your successes. Choose to believe in yourself and your abilities. Give yourself the time and attention you need to live well.

Rediscover your passions.
Give yourself time to uncover what you're passionate about and find ways to make those passions a regular part of your life.

Play.
Schedule time for leisure and play. Let yourself enjoy time off—it's good for your health!

Meaningful relationships.
Elevate and nurture meaningful relationships in your life.

Give back.
Find a way to contribute to making the world a better place.

Live in the moment and practice conscious living.
Practice being present in your life. Show up fully, live with intention, and make the moments count.

Consider for a moment that the real purpose of your life is to be fully involved in living. The preceding exercises will allow you to be present for the journey and fully embrace it. I believe if you strengthen your spiritual fitness, soon you will be overflowing with passion, purpose, and fulfillment. You'll feel strong and inspired to enjoy the journey into your own awesome life.

Are you ready to live a life full of purpose that makes your spirit soar? Commit. Commit to this journey. Commit to intentional living. Push through fears, resistance, and the unknown. Be comfortable being uncomfortable in the name of personal growth. Do the work and trust that the pain and challenges you encounter when developing your self are all part of the process. Put in the effort because you want the result: a deeper, more connected, meaningful life. Don't let your career, your hobbies, your responsibilities, your commitments, or your projects define who you are. You define who you are. You pour yourself into what you do. You are the work. And you are here for a one-time and one-time-only event: your life.

PART V
Balanced Body Breakthrough

Actually, I just woke up one day and decided I didn't want to feel like that anymore, or ever again. So I changed. Just like that.
—*Author unknown*

It took me about two full years to heal from burnout and achieve my vision of life balance. The first year was incredibly challenging. I worked with three separate coaches on different areas of my well-being. I remember feeling scared to spend money and take so much time to invest in myself, but I was worth every hour and every cent. Having real support and weekly scheduled time dedicated to my needs kept me accountable and moving toward my goals. Through a lot of effort, I met my challenges head-on and worked to overcome the negative thoughts and habits that prevented me from fully living my life. I'm not going to lie—it was hard. You have to be ready to be honest with yourself. You have to be ready to be vulnerable, to get uncomfortable, and to do real work to heal your life.

The first year allowed me to gain back my health, fitness, and strength. From this new foundation of wellness, I rebuilt my life according to my own definition of success. I built up my ability to stand up for my own needs, wants, and life. With a strong sense of self-worth and self-respect, I was able to draw healthy boundaries and prioritize my own needs first. These skills allowed me to shape my life and design my happiness. My moral standards changed; the new standard became my happiness—first—because in the end, happiness is simply living your life your own way, and I believe we all deserve that.

Self-care and balance require practice every day. Now that I have myself back, I think of my life as a precious gift that I don't plan to waste. I set out in this book to share my personal story, how it led me to be the spirited and balanced coach I am today. A lot has changed since that wake-up call on my studio floor. I have deep respect for the woman I am now because I fought to become her. There is an energy, strength, and life force in me now that I never dreamed possible. People often comment on my energy, vitality, power, and zest. I appreciate hearing these words because they remind me of how much I went through to get here and how much I've transformed myself, inside and out. I'm not perfect and don't ever expect to be, but "Progress is not perfection" is my slogan for powerful living.

I see so many struggle to find balance, health, and self-love. Burnout and stress are a growing epidemic that is making our world sick, tired, and joyless. My goal was to make this book a source of inspiration, information, encouragement, and support so that you don't lose yourself in the quest for worldly success. The resources in this book are real, tested, and ready to change your life. It doesn't matter what your entry point is or when your wake-up call strikes. Whether it's burnout, sickness, a breakup, addiction, injury, loss, or reading something that speaks to you, embrace it. You will find your wake-up call to be a chance to reinvent your life, live on your own terms, and find more meaning in every moment. I hope that I've shown you there are many tools in your hands to help you get back on when you fall off track and that it is possible to get your mind, body, and spirit in shape so you can love your life.

Remember: you are a work in progress, which means you get there a little at a time, not all at once. When you feel like you're running in circles, know that we all feel like that sometimes, especially when life's demands are high and the work is challenging. This doesn't mean you should give up. Adjust as needed, but keep putting one foot in front of the other. You are not really running in circles; you are running upward, gradually. The path is not a straight line but a zigzag . . . and by reading this book, you have already climbed higher than you may realize.

I want you to know you are always right where you need to be to take your next step. There's absolutely nothing about your present circumstances that prevents you from making progress. All you ever have to decide is what to do next—just the next tiniest step. You don't have to have it all figured out to take this step and move forward. Just do the best you can until you know better. Once you know better, do better.

Your journey will not be perfect, and you will mess up. But remember: mistakes and failures are the stepping-stones of growth and success. Even when something doesn't work out, it's still necessary practice—and everything takes practice. To be successful in the long run, you must fail sometimes. Don't let the fear of making the wrong decision prevent you from making any decision at all. In the end, failure is what makes you stronger and enables you to reach your goals.

Life can and will continue to be chaotic and to challenge you. But that doesn't mean that the world inside of you has to be that way too. You have everything you need to live with power, purpose, health, and wellness.

If ever you forget your own greatness, I am here to remind you of your strength. Stay committed, positive, present, and persistent. Keep going and keep growing. You are the only one who can create your happiness. The life you live is ultimately the life you choose. Make it count. This is your life, and you can choose to love it.

AFTERWORD

Hi, Caroline,

My name is Megan. I am 19 years old, and I am writing to you to say thank you. I have struggled with body image and exercise my entire life. When I was 12 years old I was extremely over weight, and by the time I was 14 I was in the beginning stages of anorexia. I went from being a kid who hated sports and loved junk food to a teenage girl who would go days without eating and exercised constantly. As I got a little older I realized that neither scenario was healthy. I cared only about my exterior and not about my health. As I started to eat again, I gained weight, which was good, but I wasn't happy with how I looked.

By age 16 I knew how to eat healthy and loved the way good, nutritious food made me feel, but I HATED exercising because I associated it with the struggles I had with my eating disorder. Again, I still hated the way I looked.

About two years ago is when I found your YouTube channel. I was looking for workouts to make me skinny while busting my butt and hating exercise. Your channel was different. Your exercises eased me into a healthy fitness regime, and your positivity, energy, and kindness made me realize that a healthy lifestyle is achievable by forgetting the exterior and, most important, having a positive outlook on yourself, others, and life.

Now I am the happiest I have ever been. I feel amazing, move every day, and eat healthy food for energy to keep me going. I would like to say you were a huge part of how I feel today. Thank you, thank you, thank you!

In health AND happiness

Megan

Megan,

I can't even begin to tell you how incredibly touched and inspired I was by your story. Thank you for taking the time to write and to share your journey so openly with me. I am extremely grateful that YouTube brought us together and allowed us to share time online being healthy, happy, and positive. Your story is exactly why I do the work I do: to help others develop a positive relationship to self and exercise that adds quality to their lives. Thank you for being part of my community. I hope to see you continue dreaming big, being brave, accomplishing goals, loving life, and loving yourself. Your letter touched my heart in a powerful way. You have truly inspired me, and I am honored to have been a part of your journey.

Your story can inspire others to adopt a healthy and happy relationship to exercise. WE are the change in the world! WE can help others live a life that FEELS good and is positive simply by doing it ourselves. Thank you for being the change and helping create a healthier, more positive, more self-loving world. I hope you know how beautiful you are inside and out. And I hope you know that your life is positively impacting the health and happiness of the planet.

Till next time—keep inspiring and keep shining. From the bottom of my heart, thank you for this beautiful note.

Caroline

Caroline,

Wow! I did not expect a response. I can truly tell you care about what you do and it makes a huge difference in the lives of others. I just thought I should say thank you, because you definitely were a part of the push I needed to get me where I am today.

I think that a healthy body image and acceptance of self are so important in creating a happier life. Thank you from the bottom of my heart. I do hope to inspire others the way you do.

Also, your YouTube channel, Facebook page, and weekly newsletters have inspired someone all the way in Canada! Good for you! :)

Megan

AUTHOR'S NOTE

Every day is a new day, filled with new possibilities. Never ever assume that you're stuck with the way things are. Life changes every second, and so can you.

I am here to cheer you on through all of life's changes. Keep going, keep growing, and stay positive, my friends.

Caroline

ACKNOWLEDGMENTS

The creation of this book has been a long-term goal that would not have been achieved without all the people who invested in the Inkshares kickstarter campaign and helped in making this product a reality. You made this dream possible, and I will always be grateful. To all of you: *We did it!* Thank you for supporting me and for helping the world live in balance.

Balanced Body Breakthrough tells part of my personal story, so it has been a pleasure to remember the many people who have touched my life personally and professionally along the path.

I am grateful to my mom for raising me in health, gratitude, and positivity. Her spirit lives on to inspire me every day. To my dad for being my rock, my leader, and my endless source of sunshine. To my brother, Tim, and his incredible wife, Amber, for teaching me how to live and love with heart. To my grandmother Joan, who is my inspiration in living a long and vibrant life. To all my family for believing in me, supporting me from all across the United States, and cheering me on throughout the ups and downs in this incredible journey of life.

So many people have helped form my career. I wouldn't be where I am today without my mentors Petra Kolber, Shannon

Fable, Erika Quest, Elisabeth Marsh, and Buddy Machua. These incredibly inspirational people have been a catalyst in helping me dream big and build a career based on my unique strengths and personal vision of success.

Special thanks to all of my friends for their unwavering support and for helping me live a balanced body life. To Jessica Wolfrom for encouraging me to "go for it" and for generously lending her eyes to edits. To Michelle McGovern, Philip Stenberg, and Britt Blum, who volunteered time to reading first drafts. To my lovely German intern, Anna Kemph, for being a positive light in my life and helping me launch the book's crowd-funding campaign. To Hanson Lenyon for his friendship and for giving me the work opportunity that forever changed the trajectory of my career. To my acupuncturist, Michelle Graves, for her talent and heart and for teaching me so much about holistic health. To coach Ashley Relf for helping me find my strength and build a balanced body. To my hairstylist, Wes Pine of Wes Pine Salon, for taking such good care of my crazy hair and helping me shine for the book images. To Mark Kuroda for his phenomenal talent, photography, creative expertise, and continual support in living a powerful life. To the staff at Lululemon and Lululemon Grant Avenue San Francisco for their community, heart, advocacy, and encouragement. Thanks also to Fitbit, EQUINOX, Tsuya Brand, ALOHA, Vega, Clearly Kombucha, and all the companies that partner with me in helping the world to live in health. Finally, to my community of clients, colleagues, and friends who join me all around the world in training for a positive life: Thank you. You are the reason I find fulfillment through my work. Sharing life with you is what keeps me going, and I love every minute of it.

ABOUT THE AUTHOR

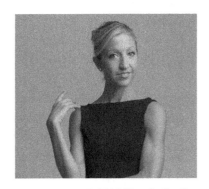

Caroline Jordan is a San Francisco–based corporate wellness consultant, fitness professional, and community spokesperson. She graduated from the University of California, Davis with a degree in Communications and Dance, and is certified by WellCoaches, the American Council on Exercise, Aerobic and Fitness Association of America, Schwinn Cycling, Balletone, and several other health and wellness agencies. Caroline has been recognized as the "Group Fitness Instructor of the Year" by UC Davis, "Group Fitness Instructor of Excellence" by EQUINOX, and as the "Personal Trainer with Passion" from the American Council on Exercise. She has been in ballet shoes since age three and hasn't stopped moving since. She is an avid runner, swimmer, cyclist, and dancer who strives to inspire others to find joy in movement.

Caroline has been a featured fitness professional in *Shape*, *SF Weekly*, *San Francisco Chronicle*, and *IDEA* and writes regularly for established wellness websites. She is a brand ambassador for Lululemon, Fitbit, ALOHA, Vega, Tsuya by Kristi Yamaguchi, and Clearly Kombucha. Caroline is a performer and personality who inspires and educates through TV, video, radio, print, and modeling productions.

Caroline leads regular classes, workshops, retreats, and seminars designed to help people keep their minds, bodies, and spirits in great shape. Her mission is to create an environment of awareness and support, inspire positive lifestyle change, and provide real resources people can immediately use to improve the quality of their lives. She believes that self-care is health care and that with the right support anyone can achieve their vision of living well and leading a healthy, happy life. Caroline works to help others to create a life that feels good on the inside and to live every moment with wisdom, well-being, and gratitude.

> *From burnout to balance. Get your mind, body, and*
> *spirit in great shape so you can love your life.*
> *Caroline*

LIST OF PATRONS

This book was made possible in part by the following grand patrons who preordered the book on inkshares.com. Thank you!

Aaron Marienthal

Alexis Marie Tiongson

Alison B. Graves

Amy Jeanette Lenz

Anna Kempf

Blake Jamieson

Brianna Haag

Carolina Marquez

Carolyn Rohde

Christi Deakin

Chris Austin

Dan Lynch

Dave Dobrow

Jennifer Marie Kirchhofer

Kristy Mikaelian

Leslie A. Zingarelli

Lisa Kant

Liz Walz

Michelle Gordon

Michelle M. Olson

Rachael Claudio

Sheri Jordan

Sabrina Kippur

Steve Chen

Suchil Samant

Weldon H. Jordan

Quill

Quill is an imprint of Inkshares, a crowdfunded book publisher. We democratize publishing by having readers select the books we publish—we edit, design, print, distribute, and market any book that meets a pre-order threshold.

Interested in making a book idea come to life? Visit inkshares.com to find new book projects or to start your own.